Vegetarianism
Movement or Moment?

Vegetarianism

Movement or Moment?

Donna Maurer

 Temple University Press
PHILADELPHIA

Temple University Press, Philadelphia 19122
Copyright © 2002 by Temple University
All rights reserved
Published 2002
Printed in the United States of America

⊛ The paper used in this publication meets the requirements of
the American National Standard for Information Sciences—Permanence
of Paper for Printed Library Materials, ANSI Z39.48-1984

Library of Congress Cataloging-in-Publication Data

Maurer, Donna, 1961–
    Vegetarianism: movement or moment? / Donna Maurer.
        p.   cm.
    Includes bibliographical references and index.
    ISBN 1-56639-935-1 (cloth : alk. paper) — ISBN 1-56639-936-X (pbk. :
alk. paper)
    1. Vegetarianism—Social aspects.   I. Title.

TX392.M417 2002
613.2′62—dc21
                                                                    2001053174

In memory of Bobbi Jo and Willow,
my dear companions for almost
fourteen years

Contents

Preface

Background

In the late 1980s, when I was studying for my master's degree at East Tennessee State University, I became interested in the sociological aspects of food and eating, in general, and vegetarianism, in particular. There were few vegetarians in northeast Tennessee back then, and during the six years that I lived in Johnson City, I think I met most of them. Teaching hatha yoga and working off and on at the local health food store, I had occasion to talk with a variety of people who were looking to adopt more balanced, healthful, and energetic lifestyles.

To the people of Johnson City—a small, close-knit community marked by political conservatism and religious fundamentalism, where social gatherings often centered on meat eating—such New Age phenomena as yoga, health foods, and vegetarianism were quite threatening, and tofu (which few people had actually tried) was a four-letter word. The people I talked with informally—at yoga classes and in the health food store—often asked me questions about vegetarian nutrition (which I was not qualified to answer); vegetarian cooking (which I could offer some advice on); and how to get along with their meat-eating families, friends, and co-workers (which I could sympathize about but offer no real answers to).

By the time I moved to Tennessee, I had spent several years as a semivegetarian, eating some fish, and then an ovo-lacto-vegetarian, consuming no meat or seafood but eating some eggs and dairy products. It was not until my stay in Johnson City, however, that I began to think about the social process of becoming a vegetarian. As is true for most vegetarians, my dietary and lifestyle changes had occurred over a long time, with several influences affecting my choices. As an undergraduate at the University of Massachusetts at Dartmouth, I had explored everything that I perceived to be radical. And during this period, about three years had passed between the time I stopped eating red meat and the time I first called myself a vegetarian. My roommates and I belonged to the local food co-op in New Bedford, and for the first time, I started to think about the origins of some of what I was eating. As a lifelong animal lover, I began to find the meat on my plate disgusting. And like many new vegetarian wanna-bes, I compensated for my rejection of meat by eating more eggs and dairy products—never stopping to consider how these foods were produced.

My life experiences in Massachusetts and Tennessee led me to see vegetarianism as a socially influenced personal choice— a lifestyle. I became interested in studying the process of *how* people become vegetarians, and in the late 1980s, I decided to take on this topic as a research project. Searching the social science and humanities literature for what others had written about vegetarians, I found surprisingly little. Most of the literature consisted of history journal articles on nineteenth-century vegetarian figures and vegetarian communes such as Octagon City and Fruitlands. However, I also found historian James Whorton's *Crusaders for Fitness;* Janet Barkas's *The Vegetable Passion;* and Anne Murcott's edited collection *The Sociology of Food and Eating,* which includes British sociologist Julia Twigg's "Vegetarianism and the Meanings of Meat."[1] As I continued my research, I discovered that other sociologists, in both the United States and the United Kingdom, were studying the process of becoming a vegetarian. And I learned that nutritional scientists and dietitians—several of whom were researching characteristics common among vegetarians —had conducted more research on the social aspects of vegetarianism than had the social scientists.[2]

In my early project, I outlined a typology of "processual elements" toward becoming a vegetarian that were found among the twenty-three vegetarians I interviewed. Although I focused on the experiences of these individuals, I gradually learned that there was more to vegetarianism than food, recipes, and a few significant books such as Frances Moore Lappé's *Diet for a Small Planet* and Peter Singer's *Animal Liberation*.[3] I began to subscribe to *Vegetarian Times* (a mass-marketed magazine), *Vegetarian Journal* (first published by the Baltimore Vegetarians, which later became the Vegetarian Resource Group [VRG]), and *FARM Report* (published by the Farm Animal Reform Movement [FARM]). Through *Vegetarian Journal* and *FARM Report*, I learned about the activities of vegetarian groups throughout the country and such national celebrations as the Great American Meat-Out (a national day of meatless eating). I found out that a vegetarian group in Knoxville had created a media stir when its members managed to persuade then governor Lamar Alexander to proclaim October 1 World Vegetarian Day. Following a flood of letters and phone calls from the meat industry, however, Alexander agreed to proclaim a World Beef Day and a World Poultry Day as well.

I began to realize that the vegetarian movement was much more than a group of people changing their eating habits. Masked by what seemed to be a dietary choice and lifestyle was an organizational structure and ideology that looked very much like a social movement: "a collectivity acting with some continuity to promote or resist a change in the society or a group of which it is a part."[4] My rethinking of vegetarianism led to the research project on which this book is based.

In an effort to find out everything I could about the organization of vegetarian activities, I subscribed to every publication put out by (and requested additional information from) every group I came across that appeared to be a vegetarian organization or an animal rights organization that in

some way promoted vegetarianism. I narrowed the field of national vegetarian organizations to seven, and I set out to interview not only leaders of these groups but also other longtime vegetarian activists not directly associated with the
organizations. To find out about local vegetarian groups, I
prepared an open-ended questionnaire, which was answered
by ninety-seven active groups, many of whom also sent me
complimentary copies of their newsletters. In addition, I par-
ticipated in local vegetarian group activities in Connecticut
and New York. And between 1995 and 1999, I attended several regional and national conferences—mostly to observe but
also occasionally to speak about my work in order to gain
feedback. (See Appendix A for a more detailed description of
my research methodology.)

During my research, I moved from an ovo-lacto-vegetarian diet to a vegan diet and lifestyle (consuming and wearing
no animals or animal by-products). I had tried to become a
vegan several times over the years, but I had given in each
time, either to hunger when I was traveling or to the use of
my warm woolen coats during the winter. Before I began my
research, I decided to make an effort once again to become a
vegan. In part, I was motivated by my own convictions, but I
also wanted to experience the daily trials and tribulations that
vegans typically encounter. As a result, I stopped eating eggs
and dairy products and became more attentive to "hidden"
animal ingredients such as whey and casein. I gave away my
wool and silk clothing; I replaced my leather shoes with foot-
wear made of materials such as plastic, cloth, rubber, and PVC
(polyvinyl chloride); and I began to contemplate whether bees
suffer in the honey cultivation process.

I did not succeed completely, so when I was faced with the
inevitable question from my interviewees, "Are you a vegan?"
I would reply that I was "98 percent." At that time, I still consumed some products that contained animal-derived ingredients—such as the "nondairy" creamer that I put in my cof-

fee—and I did not want to risk being viewed as insincere or disingenuous. (I have since learned to take my coffee black or with soy milk or rice milk.) Usually people responded by saying that it is impossible to be *truly* vegan—that, in the course of daily life, one cannot avoid consuming or using products that contain some animal-derived ingredients. Almost any magazine or newspaper, for example, contains photographs produced with the animal-derived ingredient gelatin.

Like many social scientists who study issues close to their hearts, I chose to research the vegetarian movement because I care about its key issues; I am a sympathizer—and to some extent, a participant. And like other sympathizing sociologists, I necessarily find myself revealing in this book some of what I perceive as the movement's negative or unproductive aspects. At times I feel uncomfortable presenting criticisms, even though my interpretations have evolved out of close observation and careful reflexive thought. Still, my sympathy with the movement only strengthens my commitment to presenting a study that is useful to the movement's leaders and participants. In addition, as a sociologist, I want my work not only to contribute to an understanding of how social movements function but also, finally, to make sure that vegetarianism is placed on the map of social movements.

Plan of the Book

To understand the vegetarian movement, we need some background: Why and how do people become vegetarians? Is vegetarianism becoming more popular? Is it a fad or a trend? What are its historical roots in North America? Do health professionals view vegetarian diets as healthful or unhealthful? To give a sense of vegetarianism's place in contemporary society, Chapters 1 and 2 explore these and other questions. Although people become vegetarians for a variety of reasons, in the United States and Canada, most vegetarians are motivated by a desire for self-improvement—a desire to be healthier and more energetic.[5] Rooted in this motivation, the North American vegetarian movement boasts historical figures such as Sylvester Graham, William Andrus Alcott, Ellen G. White, and John Harvey Kellogg, who have promoted vegetarian diets as the panacea for ills that result from an increasingly industrialized and chaotic world. Today most vegetarian organizations continue to focus on promoting the health aspects of vegetarianism, an approach that taps into popular concerns. For a variety of reasons that are explored in the early chapters of this book, however, this focus has made it difficult to generate the resources necessary for conducting large-scale campaigns or for directly confronting the meat industry.

Chapter 3 begins our look at the structure and organization of the vegetarian movement. In addition to considering the many different types of vegetarian organizations that contribute to movement activities (both throughout the United States and Canada and within local communities), this chapter considers the role of other interests—particularly the animal rights, health food, and environmental movements— in supporting vegetarian principles. Chapter 3 also looks at whether the meat industry, in its role as a countermovement, helps or hinders the efforts of the vegetarian cause.

Chapter 4 examines the idea that the vegetarian ideology plays a crucial role in how movement members choose and implement strategies for change and discusses the ways that different organizations articulate the vegetarian ideology. This chapter presents the different tenets of vegetarianism—compassion for animals, concern for the environment, and the healthful aspects of a vegetarian diet—and (as an introduction to some of the key internal issues that the vegetarian movement currently faces) considers recent challenges to the definition of the term "vegetarian."

Although, like other social movements, the vegetarian movement uses various strategies for promoting cultural and social change, perhaps to a greater degree than some, it focuses on encouraging change among individuals. Chapter 5, which considers the strategies of the vegetarian movement in depth, highlights the fact that these strategies are based on leaders' assumptions about how personal, cultural, and social changes occur.

Chapter 6 focuses on an important strategic dilemma of the vegetarian movement: how to develop a collective identity among participants without alienating potential new recruits. Here we examine how the movement's efforts to reach a broad audience by focusing on health issues affect the ability of participants to achieve a collective identity.

The role of vegetarian organizations has included not only providing support for those who choose a vegetarian lifestyle but also working to increase the availability of vegetarian foods in grocery stores, restaurants, hospitals, schools, and workplaces. Clearly, by any measure, vegetarian specialty items such as veggie dogs, veggie burgers, soy milk, and tofu have become increasingly accessible, and growing numbers of people—including nonvegetarians—have been trying and even demanding them. The sale of vegetarian foods has steadily increased since the late 1980s, with the market for these items ballooning from $138 million in 1989 to an estimated $662 million in 1999,[6] providing new money-making opportunities for food producers, distributors, and restaurateurs. In its exploration of this new market, Chapter 7 examines the potential effects on both the growth of the vegetarian movement and the public's acceptance of vegetarian diets.

The final chapter of this book assesses the current status of and the future possibilities for the vegetarian movement: Is the movement doomed to marginality? Will we see an increase in the number of vegetarians, or will we see merely an increase in the number of people who occasionally enjoy meatless meals? And what exactly would constitute success for the vegetarian movement? In addition, this chapter looks at how the analysis herein is applicable to other social movements: What can we learn from examining the vegetarian movement? What can we ascertain about other social movements—such as the animal rights and environmental movements—that promote lifestyle change in an effort to produce cultural change? Are some strategies likely to be more successful than others? Chapter 8 brings the book to a close by considering the impact that the vegetarian movement has had on society and the relevance of this study to understanding similar causes.

In light of the fact that the North American vegetarian movement has persisted for nearly two centuries, it is surprising that it has escaped sociological analysis until now. In part, this can be explained by the fact that—on the surface—the movement seems more like an aggregate of people who are changing their eating habits than an organized effort for change. The following chapters take us beneath these surface appearances and open the way for an exploration of the movement and its cultural impact.

Acknowledgments

Many people involved in the vegetarian movement contributed to this project by participating in interviews, completing surveys, responding to requests for information, and providing information about their groups' activities. Others, many of whom I do not even know by name, influenced how I shaped this work in more subtle ways—through casual conversations at meetings and conferences. I express my deep appreciation to each and every person who talked to and corresponded with me.

This project could never have taken form without a dissertation fellowship from Southern Illinois University (1995–1996) and a postdoctoral fellowship from the John S. Knight Writing Program at Cornell University (1998–1999). In addition, my friends and colleagues at these institutions provided the support I needed to move my study to completion.

Several people encouraged, inspired, and helped me directly or indirectly: Michael Ames, Thomas Burger, Marilyn D'Antonino, Richard Lanigan, Otto Maurer, Donald McKinley, Mareena McKinley-Wright, Calvin Moore, Kelley Raab, Sandi Rodriquez, Jeffery Sobal, Bill Walsh, Rhys Williams, and Peter Wissoker. I also owe special thanks to Joel Best, who guided and inspired me at every stage of this project.

Vegetarianism
Movement or Moment?

1 What Is Vegetarianism? And Who Are the Vegetarians?

> Is vegetarianism a social movement? To most of us, it would seem that it is, but it is also different from other social movements. It is not a social movement like civil rights or women's suffrage, because the *primary* objective of those seeking to promote vegetarianism is not political. One could certainly make political demands on the basis of vegetarianism . . . but attitudes towards food are deeper than laws or politics; they are felt literally and figuratively at the "gut level."
> —Keith Akers, "Out of Synch?"

What is vegetarianism? Is it a diet or a lifestyle? Is it a social movement or a bunch of people who happen to eat the same way? Is it a passing fad or a developing trend?

When meat eaters hear the term "vegetarian," they typically think of an ovo-lacto-vegetarian, someone who eats no meat, poultry, or fish but who consumes some dairy products and eggs. But there are also lacto-vegetarians, who eat dairy products but not eggs; ovo-vegetarians, who consume eggs but not dairy products; and vegans, who consume (and wear) no animal products or by-products whatsoever. And then there are those who call themselves vegetarians even though they occasionally eat meat or seafood. These definitions of vegetarianism suggest that it is simply a dietary preference that requires adherence to no particular ideology.

1

For many people, however, being a vegetarian means more than following a set of dietary proscriptions—it is a way of life. Although there are those who eliminate meat from their diets for economic reasons, these individuals typically return to meat eating as they gain the financial means to do so.[1] For these "hardship vegetarians," meatless eating is neither a desirable nor a completely free choice. People who become vegetarians by choice, however, typically use diet as a form of self-expression and creativity.[2] Vegetarians, for example, frequently explore new foods, shop at food co-ops and natural food stores, and peruse vegetarian cookbooks and magazines for new recipes. They often discuss their food choices with family, and friends, and, to varying degrees, they incorporate vegetarianism into their self-concepts.

Is the vegetarian movement, then, simply an aggregate of people practicing the same lifestyle? After all, vegetarians do not appear to be particularly politically active or publicly outspoken, most do not belong to any movement or organization, and national campaigns promoting vegetarianism are rare. Still, behind the appearance of arbitrary adherence to a common lifestyle exists a structured set of organizations, ideas, and related phenomena: a movement that includes local and national organizations, a body of movement literature, a set of relatively coherent arguments, and a wide range of products and services. A vegetarian ideology—vegetarianism—provides both a critique of meat eating and the vision of a vegetarian world. The vast majority of vegetarians draw from this ideology to express their personal motivations for adopting this lifestyle.[3]

Vegetarian organizations, despite their lack of public visibility, are the backbone of the vegetarian way of life: Here agendas are set, vocabulary and other symbols are defined, and information and networking services are made available. These organizations create and distribute literature about the meaning of vegetarianism and hold meetings and conferences to celebrate vegetarian lifestyles. Vegetarian groups are central to movement activities because they generate and promote ideas about the most effective ways to achieve personal, cultural, and social change—in other words, how to be a vegetarian and how to create a vegetarian world. Although many people (including many social scientists) perceive vegetarianism as an individual phenomenon, the significance of vegetarian organizations points to its *social* dimension.

But is vegetarianism a fad or a trend? Interest groups such as the National Cattlemen's Beef Association argue that vegetarian diets are a passing fad, bound to go in and out of style like bell bottoms, new-wave music, and mood rings. Other food industry watchers have called vegetarianism one of the "top 10 trends to watch and work on," particularly among teenagers and college students, and the National Restaurant Association has identified vegetarian foods as the wave of the future.[4] The American Dietetic Association (ADA), the U.S. Department of Agriculture (USDA), the National Institute of Nutrition in Canada, and Dietitians of Canada have all given scientific legitimacy to the mainstreaming of vegetarianism by declaring well-planned vegetarian diets to be nutritious and healthful.[5] Although vegetarianism's popularity has waxed and waned—with its peaks occurring in the mid-1800s and in the 1960s and early 1970s—it has held a small but consistent following in the United States and Canada since the 1820s.

Why Do People Become Vegetarians?

People have articulated a variety of reasons for adopting vegetarian diets: personal health, concern about the treatment of farm animals (which often includes belief in animal rights), environmental issues, world hunger concerns, and disgust at the thought of consuming the flesh of a dead animal.[6] Often vegetarians, and those who study them, use a simpler dichotomy: health reasons and ethical (or moral) reasons.[7] In

North America, most people begin the path to vegetarianism for health reasons. For example, in a 1992 poll that the market research company Yankelovich, Clancy, Shulman conducted for *Vegetarian Times* magazine, 46 percent of the 601 self-described vegetarians surveyed cited health as the most important reason for becoming a vegetarian, 15 percent cited animal welfare, and 12 percent cited the influence of family and friends. Others cited ethical reasons (5 percent) and the environment (4 percent), and 18 percent checked the category "not sure/other."[8] Often, concern about dietary fat prompts the move toward vegetarianism,[9] though concern about the safety of the meat supply, the desire to lose weight, and holistic treatment plans to help prevent or improve medical conditions such as cancer and heart disease can also inspire the move.

For some people, the sources of motivation change or increase as they adopt vegetarian diets. Most commonly, a person initially becomes motivated by health issues and gradually adopts ethical reasons as well.[10] For example, as a woman in her fifties explained, she originally decided to cut down on her consumption of red meat because she was concerned about chemical contamination. Later, her work with primates led to an interest in the animal rights movement: "The process all started when I became aware of how contaminated the foods were. [I] always cared about animals, but I think it started with contamination. And the more I read about contamination, the more I realized what was being done to the animals. And I guess it was in the late 60s. So it took a good 10, 15 years before I really got primed."[11] For most, becoming a vegetarian is a gradual process that involves reading vegetarian literature, talking with other vegetarians, and defending their lifestyle to others. This social interaction facilitates the process of learning about vegetarianism.

This move from a single motivation to multiple motivations for adopting a vegetarian diet tends to strengthen the commitment to vegetarianism. This increased commitment can, in turn, lead to social activism. Though their hierarchy of reasons can shift over time, at some point most leaders of vegetarian organizations incorporate an ethical motivation into the mix. For example, Francis Janes, a long-time EarthSave International leader, became ethically motivated after he viewed a video based on John Robbins's *Diet for a New America:*[12]

> I think if you ask today what my motivations are to live my lifestyle, health would be just a bonus now. For me, if someone told me today, if you came up to me with confirmed medical evidence that said, "Being a vegetarian has no medical or health benefits," I would say to you, "I'm so clear about the ethical and the environmental benefits of doing this that it doesn't matter." I would still follow the path. And so your whole perspective on what brought you to this path in the first place and why you do it today . . . does shift and change.[13]

Even those leaders who are initially inspired by ethical issues are likely to embrace multiple motivations along the way. For many vegetarians—and particularly for organization leaders—"being" a vegetarian is not a static state; it is a process of "becoming" through shifting personal motivations and increasing degrees of commitment.

People who become motivated by ethical issues are more likely than others to become vegans, those who abandon the consumption of all animal products and by-products. In fact, the ethical orientations of most vegetarian movement leaders—which are usually related to concerns about animal suffering and the deleterious effects of meat production on the environment—have led the vast majority to follow a vegan lifestyle. For example, Stacey Vicari, former president of EarthSave International, reports that her commitment to the elimination of animal suffering helps her to maintain her vegan lifestyle: "When I read *Diet for a New America* what influenced me the most was the animal section of the book. And for me that's what's given me the perseverance to really stay true to a vegan diet. There are days within my vegan diet that I'll eat fatty popcorn at the movie theater or that I'll eat vegan carrot cake at a party. But I don't eat cheese, and I don't eat ice cream, and I don't eat meat, because I have strong convictions."[14] Commitment to animal welfare or rights and to the environment, which helps vegans to maintain their lifestyle (particularly in situations where deviation from social expectations draws negative reactions from others), is manifested in the willingness of vegetarian leaders to sacrifice their time, energy, and other resources in the promotion of vegetarianism.

How Do People Become Vegetarians?

Although there are some who make an abrupt change to vegetarianism, most people become vegetarians gradually. The most common path to vegetarianism is to eliminate red meat from the diet; then poultry; then seafood; and, for some, then eggs and dairy products.[15] This progression seems to reflect a commonly held set of beliefs about both the health hazards of these foods and the amount of suffering to animals that their consumption causes.[16] People who abruptly "go vegan," on the other hand, are more likely to be motivated by ethical concerns or to have experienced extreme disgust over the consumption of meat.[17]

The process of becoming a vegetarian usually involves social interaction with someone who already practices vegetarianism, often a family member or friend but sometimes merely an appealing acquaintance.[18] In one study, 63 percent of vegetarians surveyed claimed that their decision had been influenced by other vegetarians; among the same respondents, 40 percent claimed that they had influenced the decision of at least one other vegetarian.[19] Social contact can be especially motivating for those who are already predisposed to vegetarianism. For example, one woman in her thirties became a vegetarian after marrying an ovo-lacto-vegetarian who both inspired her and provided the support she needed. As she explains, "Well, it was [my husband who motivated me]. . . . I already had strong leanings toward [vegetarianism] to begin with and I guess I never had that extra little push to do it and also didn't quite know how to go about it. . . . And in talking with him, I realized how this was something I really wanted to do."[20] Established vegetarians provide both emotional support (empathizing with the difficulties that new vegetarians sometimes encounter) and instrumental support (offering information about how to prepare new foods and where to shop).[21]

Although many new vegetarians are strongly influenced by social interaction, some are motivated by books (and even films) that deal with vegetarian issues.[22] Prominent books such as Frances Moore Lappé's 1971 *Diet for a Small Planet,* Peter Singer's 1975 *Animal Liberation,* John Robbins's 1987 *Diet for a New America,* and Erik Marcus's 1998 *Vegan: The New Ethics of Eating,* for example, all address issues regarding hunger and animal suffering.[23] This suggests that people who are influenced more by media than by social interaction may be motivated more by ethics than by personal health concerns.

In the course of adopting vegetarianism, some people (particularly those without other vegetarian social networks) find social and instrumental support in vegetarian organizations. As vegetarian advocate Keith Akers writes, "It is hard to take a 'radical' step such as rejecting meat consumption when you are completely alone in your beliefs, when none of your family or friends are vegetarians, and others regard you as part of the lunatic fringe as a consequence of your diet."[24] Local vegetarian groups throughout the United States and Canada meet—usually monthly—to enjoy potluck meals and to share recipes and other information. Vegetarian organizations also reinforce vegetarian norms—sometimes so strongly that they cause people to feel guilty about straying from their vegetarian diets.[25] Clearly, friends, family, acquaintances, and associations can greatly influence a person's choice to adopt and continue to follow a vegetarian lifestyle.

Who Is Most Likely to Become a Vegetarian?

Food consumption patterns are associated with social class, ethnicity, and gender. A profile of those who are most likely to decrease meat consumption and become vegetarians indicates white, middle-class females. Vegetarians share characteristics such as being less likely than the general population to participate in conventional religions and being more likely to consider themselves liberal and to practice health-conscious behaviors. It is not clear, however, whether these are predisposing characteristics that might influence a person to practice vegetarianism or merely consequences of engaging in a vegetarian lifestyle.

Vegetarianism and Socioeconomic Status

People who choose to follow vegetarian diets overwhelmingly hail from the middle class. Although the cost of a nutritionally sound meatless diet can rival the cost of a meat-based diet, people from lower-income groups rarely become vegetarians by choice. Instead, as those with lower socioeconomic status become upwardly mobile, they tend to increase food spending, with a large portion of this additional expenditure going toward the purchase of meat.[26] The capacity to purchase unlimited quantities of meat is associated with higher socioeconomic status. People from lower-income groups rarely become vegetarians before they acquire the capacity to purchase all of the meat (i.e., the status) they want.

People with higher socioeconomic status, in contrast, may adopt vegetarian diets in part to differentiate themselves from other social groups.[27] According to cultural historian Margaret Visser, "Modern people in rich societies have reached a stage of satiety, of exhaustion with 'choice,' that sometimes makes them want to have something they can reject."[28] Adopting a vegetarian diet helps to structure choices and generate satisfaction, and by providing a comfortable set of rules, it can contribute to one's self-concept. In their 1981 study of vegetarians and gourmets, sociologists Kurt Back and Margaret Glasgow conclude that although both groups typically consist of people from middle-class backgrounds, their food choices represent different self-concepts: "Gourmets try to integrate a large, fluid, cosmopolitan middle-class culture, and vegetarians define themselves negatively and create strong boundaries against the general society."[29] Vegetarians may create these strong boundaries by identifying with rules that set them apart from others. The desire to follow a structured set of norms—thus alleviating tension generated by a proliferation of choices and enhancing one's status identification as "different" from others—is most likely to occur among people from the middle and upper socioeconomic classes. These groups have less interest than those from lower-income groups in holding onto meat's generally accepted status as a representation of power, prestige, and strength.

Vegetarianism and Ethnicity

Although the relationship between ethnicity and vegetarianism is not well understood, ethnicity may play a role in the likelihood that a person will adopt this lifestyle. One survey reports that 1 percent of African Americans "never eats poultry,"[30] which suggests that no more than 1 percent is vegetarian. Given the survey's margin of error, moreover, the actual number could be a mere fraction of a percent. There are no other surveys of the general population on record that address ethnicity with regard to vegetarianism. It is certainly possible, however—and perhaps even likely—that certain ethnic groups, particularly various Asian groups, practice vegetarianism in higher percentages than do blacks or even whites. Based on my observation at vegetarian conferences and my conversations with organization leaders, I would estimate that people of color constitute less than 5 percent of group membership and conference participants.

The predominance of white vegetarians might be explained by arguing that the relevant independent variable is socioeconomic class rather than race. Given the income discrepancy between whites and ethnic minorities (and the desirability of beef), we might expect ethnic minorities (as a social group) to value meat (and especially beef) highly. These factors suggest that as ethnic minorities at the lowest income levels (just like whites at the lowest income levels) become upwardly mobile, they are likely to consume more beef.

Group differences in income offer only a partial explanation, however. People's adherence to traditional ethnic foodways, which often include meat, may also explain why people of color are unlikely to become vegetarians. People adhere to ethnic foodways (or altered and updated versions of these foodways) in order to maintain ties with their cultural heritages,[31] and they often do so with little conscious effort. A person learns food values by "copying . . . attitudes and behaviors from those with whom [he or she] identifies."[32] Because these values become habituated through practice, many nutritional scientists and health promoters have complained that food habits are extremely resistant to change. People may even associate powerful early experiences with memories of food smells, tastes, and textures.[33] Following traditional ethnic foodways, moreover, can be more than simply a habit; it can be a conscious decision as well. Current trends that celebrate cultural diversity and thus encourage people to explore their culinary roots may well lead them away from vegetarianism.

Vegetarianism and Gender

Surveys generally concur that close to 70 percent of all vegetarians are female[34] and that more women than men try to eat more healthfully by ceasing or reducing their consumption of red meat.[35] Historically and cross-culturally, women consume less meat than do the men in their households, especially when meat is scarce.[36] Carol Adams writes that, for men, "Meat is King": A man attains the attributes of masculinity by consuming meat, in a sort of homeopathic transfiguration in which a dead animal's former strength animates the consumer. Because vegetarian men, by definition, challenge conventional masculinity norms, they become the targets of taunts that they are not "real men."[37]

Foods often connote masculinity and femininity. For example, in many cultures, light-colored foods that have a light taste are defined as feminine, and dark-colored foods that have a heavy taste are defined as masculine.[38] Eating lightly is also commonly associated with femininity,[39] and maintaining a low-fat diet is associated with "being more attractive, intelligent, conscientious, and calm."[40] These perceptions reinforce different norms of meat consumption for men and women. However, regardless of whether women heed these food connotations, because women are typically more concerned than men about losing weight, they are more likely to diminish or eliminate heavier (usually red) meats from their diets.

Married life has deterred some women from becoming vegetarians. Some have faced spousal disapproval, rejection, and even violence.[41] As traditional household divisions of labor persist, women—both vegetarian and nonvegetarian—remain primarily responsible for the purchase and preparation of their families' food.[42] Although women often act as gatekeepers of consumption, influencing what other family members eat, hierarchical divisions of power within the family can undermine this control. Women are most likely to purchase and prepare foods, but in some cases their husbands dictate their choices. Nicki Charles and Marilyn Kerr suggest that men in families tend to have primary control over what is consumed at home, and when men are absent, children take control. Husbands may assert their control by telling their wives what to buy, refusing to eat what they prepare, or—in the most extreme cases—reacting violently when their wives refuse to prepare what they demand. Perhaps not surprisingly, then, vegetarians are less likely than the general population to be married.[43] Some women, however—both vegetarians and nonvegetarians—eat different foods from those that they prepare for their families.

Because women are socialized to base decisions on feelings of empathy rather than on logical, analytical thinking, they may tend to be more moved by vegetarianism's ethic of compassion toward animals than are men.[44] Whereas men are socialized to make moral judgments based on an effort not to interfere with the rights of other humans, women are socialized to make judgments based on a sense of responsibility to alleviate "real and recognizable trouble" in the world.[45] Therefore, women may become concerned about animal suffering as a "real trouble," and men may become concerned about a farmer's right to raise animals for food and a hunter's right to shoot deer. And women, having experienced more oppression as a group than men, may be more amenable to an egalitarian ideology that would generate more concern for animal rights. Women, more than men, are likely to be moved by vegetarian movement messages that evoke concerns for health, empathy, and compassion.[46]

Vegetarianism and Other Characteristics

Although people often associate vegetarianism with religions such as Hinduism, Buddhism, and Seventh Day Adventism, according to one study, 90 percent of vegetarians are not motivated by religion, and vegetarians are much less likely than are nonvegetarians to practice a traditional religion. At the same time, vegetarians often perceive themselves as being spiritually oriented and are more likely than the general population to engage in practices such as meditation and yoga. In my 1989 study of vegetarians in northeast Tennessee, an area with a particularly high rate of religious participation, only one out of twenty-three participants belonged to a conventional church.[47] Many of the people I interviewed in that study articulated a more individual spirituality, sometimes connected with nature. I noted comments such as the following:

> I'm very spiritual, but [I have] no particular religion. In fact I feel that religion takes us away from close communication with God.

> I'd say I'm not religious, but I'm spiritual. My father is a minister, a Baptist minister, so I've always had Christianity around to choose from. . . . I'm a pagan at heart.

> I don't go to church, but I basically go to my own church, which is outside.

For some people, vegetarianism may be an integral part of an individual spiritual ethic. At the same time, vegetarianism may—in part—replace some of the needs that religion fills for others. In particular, vegetarianism offers a perceptual framework that organizes one's personal social world, what sociologist Peter Berger calls a nomos: a schema that both generates meaning and structures choices,[48] protecting a person from chaos in the social world.

Vegetarians are no more likely than the general population to be politically active, although they may be more likely to describe themselves as liberal and less likely to adhere to such "traditional values" as obedience and adherence to the social order.[49] Vegetarians also tend to practice some health behaviors that are significantly different from those of the general population: They are less likely to consume alcohol and smoke cigarettes than are nonvegetarians.[50] And they tend to read more books about nutrition and score higher on the USDA's Healthy Eating Index of nutrition knowledge and healthful eating.[51]

Despite the various characteristics that vegetarians tend to share in common, it is important to note that there are probably more differences than similarities among vegetarians. Although more vegetarians hail from the middle class than from any other socioeconomic group, for example, vegetarians range from the wealthy to the impoverished. And although relatively few African Americans become vegetarians, Martin Luther King Jr.'s son Dexter is among those who have done so as part of a commitment to peace and social justice. And, finally, although vegetarians are typically quite health conscious, there are vegetarians who eat junk food, never exercise, and use illicit drugs. Vegetarians as a group are rather dissimilar; their one universally shared interest is a concern about the consumption of meat.

How Many Vegetarians Are There?

Given the increasing acceptance of vegetarian diets, the publicity surrounding such health hazards as E. (*Escherichia*) *coli* and *Salmonella* bacteria in meat, and the general public's fear of fat, we might expect per capita meat consumption to decrease and the percentage of the population who follow vegetarian diets to increase. Neither, however, seems to be the case. People today, on average, consume more meat, poultry, and seafood than they did in 1970. The total per capita meat, poultry, and seafood consumption rose from 177 pounds in

1970 to 192 pounds in 1997, and the USDA predicts that overall meat consumption will continue on an upward trend.[52] The typical U.S. diet has been consistently meat based; it is only the *type* of meat that has gradually shifted—from pork to beef and now from beef to poultry.

Pricing is a factor that typically affects consumers' food choices. Until refrigerated railway transportation was readily available, for example, the cost of beef reflected the high cost of transporting beef into urban areas. Because pigs could be raised inexpensively in areas close to cities,[53] the cost of pork was considerably less than the cost of beef. Until the twentieth century, therefore, pork dominated the meat market. Economists have demonstrated how various price changes have affected more recent meat consumption. Between 1960 and 1970, for example, poultry consumption rose significantly (44 percent) as prices fell; at the same time, the consumption of pork remained relatively constant as prices increased only slightly. Beef consumption in the United States rose dramatically between 1920 and 1976, declined slowly between 1976 and 1993 as beef prices increased, and started to rise slowly again in 1994.[54] Because current predictions indicate an impending decline in beef prices, some agricultural economists suggest that beef consumption will increase. Per capita figures suggest that although some people are choosing, for a variety of reasons, to eliminate or diminish their consumption of beef, those who do eat beef are eating more of it.

As noted previously, per capita meat consumption does not seem to be decreasing, and the percentage of the adult population that practices vegetarianism does not seem to be increasing substantially either. Surveys suggest that vegetarians probably constitute between 1 and 2.5 percent of the Canadian and U.S. populations.[55] Although a small percentage of the population follows some form of ovo-lacto-vegetarian or vegan diet, the number of semivegetarians is much greater:

Between six and nine million adults who claim to be vegetarians eat meat or seafood occasionally.[56]

It is difficult to know for sure how many people practice vegetarianism in the United States and Canada for two main reasons: First, taking the statistical margin of error of the survey results into account can increase or decrease the nationwide percentage of vegetarians by up to 4 percent. Second, the phrasing of survey questions affects estimates of the number of vegetarians. Several surveys ask simply, "Are you a vegetarian?" The fact that many more people identify as vegetarians than adhere to the standard definition inflates survey results. Recent surveys that tally the number of vegetarians by using self-definition indicate that the portion of the population claiming to be vegetarian rose from about 2 percent in 1980 to about 7 percent in the 1992 and 1993 (see Table 1). Surveys that tally their numbers by asking people which foods they have eliminated from their diets (meat, poultry, seafood, milk, eggs) indicate much lower numbers of vegetarians (see Table 2).[57]

From 1992 to the year 2000, between 1 and 2.5 percent of the U.S. population followed a vegetarian diet on a regular basis, and about three times as many people identified as vegetarians. Unfortunately, because we do not have the data to trace the numbers of vegetarians throughout the decades, we have no way of knowing to what degree the vegetarian population has increased or decreased over time. Existing studies do show, however, that the percentage of adult vegetarians has not changed *dramatically*. The 1994 and 1997 Roper Polls conducted for VRG suggest that the vegetarian population did not grow rapidly in the mid-1990s; the 2000 National Zogby Poll, also conducted for VRG, demonstrates an increase so small that it is unclear whether it represents an actual change or a statistical anomaly (information about the Zogby Poll is available on the VRG website—see Appendix B).[58]

All of these results reflect only the practices of U.S. adults. Even less is known about the percentage of children and teens

Table 1   Number of Adult Vegetarians in the United States,
Based on Self-Definition

Year	Who Conducted the Study	% of U.S. Adult Population
1980	U.S. Economic Research Service	2.0
1985	*American Health* magazine	3.7
1986	*Vegetarian Times* magazine	8.2
1991	Gallup (for National Restaurant Association)	5.0
1992	Yankelovich, Clancy, Shulman	7.0
1993	Thomas Dietz et al.	7.0

Sources: Adapted from Judy Jones Putnam and Lawrence A. Duewer, "U.S. Per Capita Food Consumption: Record High Meat and Sugars in 1994," *Food Review* 18, no. 2 (1995): 2–11; Joel Gurin, "Are You a Semi-vegetarian?" *American Health* (July–August 1985): 37–43; Andis Robeznieks, "How Many Are There?" *Vegetarian Times* (October 1986): 16–17; "Survey Shows Interest in Vegetarian Items," *Restaurants USA* 11, no. 8 (1991): 20–21; Judy Krizmanic, "Here's Who We Are," *Vegetarian Times* (October 1992): 72–80; Thomas Dietz et al., "Values and Vegetarianism: An Exploratory Analysis," *Rural Sociology* 60, no. 3 (1995): 533–542.

Table 2   Number of Adult Vegetarians in the United States,
Based on Operationalized Definition*

Year	Who Conducted the Study	% of U.S. Adult Population
1992	Yankelovich, Clancy, Shulman	2.3
1993	Thomas Dietz et al.	1.5
1994	Roper (for Vegetarian Resource Group)	1.0
1997	Roper (for Vegetarian Resource Group)	1.0
2000	Zogby (for Vegetarian Resource Group)	2.5

*Survey results count as vegetarians only those who state that they do not eat meat, poultry, and seafood.

Sources: Adapted from Judy Krizmanic, "Here's Who We Are," *Vegetarian Times* (October 1992): 72–80; Thomas Dietz et al., "Values and Vegetarianism: An Exploratory Analysis," *Rural Sociology* 60, no. 3 (1995): 533–542; Charles Stahler, "How Many Vegetarians Are There?" *Vegetarian Journal* 12, no. 5 (1997): 21–22; Vegetarian Resource Group, "How Many Vegetarians Are There?" (2000), accessed on-line: www.vrg.org/journal/vj2000may/2000maypoll.htm

who practice vegetarianism. According to the VRG 2000 Zogby Poll, 2 percent of youths ages six to seventeen claim that they never eat meat, fish, or poultry, and another survey reports that almost 37 percent of teens claim that they avoid eating red meat. A survey sponsored by the Physicians' Committee for Responsible Medicine (PCRM) found that 11 percent of women between ages eighteen and twenty-four "say they avoid meat, poultry, and fish."[59] Further evidence suggests that college students are particularly likely to lean toward vegetarianism; about 15 percent select a vegetarian dining hall option on any given day.[60]

Marketing professionals most commonly describe teen vegetarianism as a trend rather than a fad. According to the head of a consulting firm that markets to youths, "Among young people today, the term vegetarian reflects someone who is health-aware, health-educated, and eating in a modern, maybe even a trendy way. . . . It's become a positive label, a positive statement about yourself."[61] Another marketing group identifies veganism as a top "street trend" in alternative youth culture.[62] Without longitudinal studies, however, we can know neither whether the numbers of child and teenage vegetarians are increasing nor whether the current "trend" of teenage vegetarianism will translate into more adult vegetarians in the future. As Sally Clinton, founder of the Vegetarian Education Network, states, "Many parents think vegetarianism is just copy-cat behavior mimicking the actions of the cool kids. But those people tend to drop out of the movement within a year or so. When it's based in ethics, you stick with it."[63] The motivation behind their vegetarianism may be the key to whether the teenage vegetarians of today become the adult vegetarians of tomorrow.

Why Don't More People Become Vegetarians?

Many people regard a low-fat, high-fiber semivegetarian diet as optimal,[64] but only a small percentage of the population follows a diet that includes no meat or seafood and far fewer consume no animal products at all. With vegetarian diets increasingly being viewed as healthful and desirable, then, why do relatively few people identify as vegetarians and even fewer actually follow a vegetarian diet?

Whereas some social movements call on participants to change for the benefit of a collective good, others—such as the vegetarian movement—encourage participants to change for their own individual benefit. By using a distinction first made by sociologist Max Weber,[65] we might call the first type ethical movements and the second type exemplary movements. Ethical movements offer prescriptions for moral attitudes, whereas exemplary movements offer suggestions and general direction. In an ethical movement, adherence to prescribed rules is viewed as a duty, a moral obligation; in an exemplary movement, this adherence is a more processual, less absolute path. A social movement may include characteristics of both types, or it may evolve from one type into the other.

Vegetarian organizations often avoid presenting the public with the ethical basis for rejecting meat. Instead, they tend to take a more exemplary than ethical approach, encouraging change for one's own personal benefit. The most common strategy involves a slow educational process, centered first on health and gradually moving toward more overtly ideological concerns about the environment and animal rights. Movement leaders argue that because most people initially change their eating habits out of self-interest, promoting health benefits taps existing personal concerns. In addition, leaders suggest that many people initially resist dietary change and adopt vegetarianism gradually. Consequently, advocates typically avoid strategies that directly challenge deep-rooted meat-eating practices and beliefs, downplaying the vegetarian identity in favor of an approach that embraces as positive any and all movement toward a vegetarian diet.

Health-centered strategies may appeal to a relatively wide audience, but they are more likely to motivate people to try vegetarian foods or to experiment with semivegetarian diets than to motivate a cadre of committed vegetarian advocates. Most people value taste over health, and many think that meat tastes good. Convincing people that meat (including poultry and fish) is so unhealthful that they should eliminate it completely from their diets would seem a difficult, if not insurmountable, task. Although much scientific evidence demonstrates the healthful qualities of vegetarian diets, it is extremely difficult to argue convincingly that eating an occasional hamburger (or a little turkey at Thanksgiving) would have dramatic health consequences. As a result, people often move toward vegetarianism by cutting back on their consumption of meat, or they try vegetarianism briefly and then give it up.

People motivated by health concerns tend to be less committed to vegetarianism than those motivated by ethics. As a result of their 1999 study of vegetarianism among female physicians, Randall F. White, Jennifer Seymour, and Erica Frank concluded, "Those who were vegetarian for health reasons were more likely to consume animal flesh than others, implying that those with philosophical or religious motivation may tend to be dietary purists, and those with health motivations, pragmatists."[66] Health-motivated vegetarians may abandon vegetarianism for diets that include lower-fat, organic meat (and other animal product) alternatives. Ethically motivated vegetarians (especially vegans) are more likely than health-motivated vegetarians to find the consumption of meat repugnant,[67] and therefore they are less likely to be tempted by such products.

Health-motivated vegetarians are more likely than ethically motivated vegetarians to give in to social pressures. As one college student put it, "I'm basically a vegetarian, but I will eat a burger every once in a while if I'm out with friends."[68] As psychologists Paul Rozin, Maureen Markwith, and Caryn Stoess explain, health vegetarians "believe they will derive health benefits from meat avoidance, but are tempted by the aroma of meat, and are fighting the tendency to eat it. Under stress (strong hunger or problems in their lives) they are likely to succumb, and they may be looking for information that will absolve meat of its supposed health-damaging properties.

Moral vegetarians, in contrast, have the strong force of morality behind them."[69] Certainly, some vegetarians who have experienced a strong personal health benefit are unwavering in their vegetarian practice (and may even feel guilty when they eat meat), but without an ethical commitment, vegetarianism is a tenuous lifestyle vulnerable to changing personal tastes and stressful social circumstances.

It is significant that vegetarians motivated solely by self-benefit are unlikely to contribute to movement goals that help other humans, animals, and the planet. Although those motivated by self-interest may become involved in efforts to make vegetarian foods more widely available, the temptation to "free-ride" (reap the benefits of movement efforts without contributing to their success) can be powerful. People motivated by ethics, in contrast, more often stick with and expand their vegetarian practices (move from an ovo-lacto-vegetarian diet to a vegan lifestyle, for example) and contribute time, energy, and other resources to movement activities.

The North American vegetarian movement has always taken an exemplary approach, motivating people primarily to change for their own self-benefit. For more than 180 years, it has encouraged people to consider and has educated people about the benefits of a meatless diet. But its emphasis on the health benefits of vegetarianism does not seem to be attracting masses of new adherents. Although health professionals increasingly regard well-planned vegetarian diets as healthful—and movement organizations promote this fact—the percentage of the population that practices vegetarianism does not seem to be increasing substantially. In our world of seemingly infinite and relatively inexpensive food choices, it is a difficult task to persuade a significant portion of the population to eliminate a sizable segment of these choices. Is the vegetarian movement, then, forever doomed to marginality? Or can changes in the cultural environment and in movement strategies help to make vegetarianism not only culturally acceptable but also more widely practical and desirable?

2 Vegetarian Diets and the Health Professions

Historical Perspectives and Contemporary Issues

Many vegetarian diets do have certain inherent deficiencies. They are adequate only if they are supplemented with dairy and poultry products, which are necessary to meet the nutritional requirements of all age groups.
—Darla Erhard, "The New Vegetarians," 1973

Vegetarian diets are consistent with the *Dietary Guidelines for Americans* and can meet Recommended Dietary Allowances for Nutrients.
—U.S. Department of Agriculture and U.S. Department of Health and Human Services, *Nutrition and Your Health*, 1995

Although people in the nineteenth century often linked vegetarian diets with such social causes as abolition and temperance, Graham and other charismatic health leaders successfully encouraged many people to adopt vegetarian diets to cure or assuage health problems. Today, most North American vegetarians are still motivated by health concerns,[1] unlike their British counterparts, who historically and contemporarily have been more concerned with animal rights and ethics.[2] Although the reform components of the nineteenth-century North American vegetarian movement weakened over time, many individuals and groups have incorporated vegetarianism into various forms of political and social reform. For example, in 1948, John Maxwell ran for U.S. president on the Vegetarian Party ticket, which advocated the "extermination of cattle [raising] and conversion of their grazing lands to food production."[3] And in the 1996 U.S. presidential elections, both the Green Party and the Natural Law Party endorsed vegetarianism and sustainable agriculture in broad terms. Although vegetarian diets are occasionally mentioned in the political arena, however, vegetarian individuals and groups have focused more on legitimizing and publicizing the health benefits of vegetarianism than on making political demands.

Historically, health professionals have marginalized vegetarian diets, but beginning in the last quarter of the twentieth century, this attitude began to change dramatically. Because medical and nutritional scientists provide a voice of authority that structures the discourse on what constitutes healthful eating, they are important to the successful promotion of vegetarianism.[4] According to one survey, for example, 75 percent of Americans look to dietitians for "expert advice on issues of health and nutrition."[5] The support that the ADA, the American Heart Association (AHA), the American Cancer Society (ACS), and other such organizations have given to diets based on whole grains and fresh fruits and vegetables has contributed greatly to the ability of vegetarian groups to support their claims about the healthfulness of vegetarianism.[6] Although health organizations typically do not promote vegetarian diets outright (the ADA being, to some degree, an exception), their acknowledgment that a plant-based diet *can* be healthful (and perhaps even more healthful than an omnivorous diet) contributes to a more positive image than existed in the past. Still, controversy lingers about whether some segments of the population (for example, infants and teenage girls) are at risk for medical problems that stem from inadequate vegetarian nutrition.

Although vegetarianism itself is a philosophy, an ideology, most people initially approach vegetarianism as a diet. They think about what they will eat "instead of meat" and what choices they will make in a variety of social contexts. Even ethically motivated vegetarians find that nonvegetarians typically ask them questions that focus on health: Where do you get your protein? How do you take in enough iron? The North American vegetarian movement has always promoted diet as a means of bringing about self-improvement rather than as a means of achieving a public moral good, and popular discourse on health and fitness has perhaps strengthened this emphasis on contemporary vegetarianism as a personal, self-benefiting choice.

A Brief Historical Overview of Vegetarianism in the United States

Nineteenth-century vegetarian reformers argued the benefits of vegetarianism on both moral and medical grounds.[7] Like many Jacksonian movements, the vegetarian movement reacted to industrialization's encroachment into everyday life.[8] Medicine was becoming more technical, with the advent of new instruments (such as the stethoscope), inhalation anesthesia, diagnosis with reference to clinical statistics, and new medicines derived from vegetable sources. Science began to replace religion as the predominant moral paradigm.[9] And in the early 1800s, industrialization and modernization conflicted with new philosophical concepts that began to acknowledge the individual's capacity to reattune with nature and with God through independent, moral action.[10] The early vegetarian health reformers, sometimes called moral physiologists, offered a "system of everyday piety," a structure that enabled followers to live their lives as sacred acts without the dogma of conventional religion.[11]

The early vegetarian proponents melded together notions of spirituality and personal health that heralded individuals as being responsible for their own attunement with the Divine. The North American vegetarian movement is grounded in religion. William Metcalfe brought vegetarianism to the United States in 1817 when he settled in Philadelphia and founded the Bible Christian Church (1817–1922). Although Metcalfe spoke primarily to his congregation, he reached wider audiences through lectures and pamphlets that focused on scriptural mandates for vegetarianism and temperance.[12]

In 1830, the Bible Christian Church hired Sylvester Graham (1794–1851) as a temperance lecturer. Graham was studying medicine in Philadelphia, and the Bible Christian teachings helped move him to incorporate a vegetarian diet into his health prescriptions. In Graham's view, all stimulation was potentially health threatening; he viewed alcohol, sex, coffee, tea, spices, and meat as especially dangerous.[13] He began a movement that reached far beyond religious congregations, turning the sacred aspects of the Bible Christian philosophy into a secular morality.

At its core, the Grahamite movement was a populist one,[14] a response to increasing industrialization and social change. The marketplace assumed primary importance in this new social order, and the hearth and home took a secondary role. Graham and others saw this shift as devastating to the growth and stability of moral character. Graham's program stressed the importance of individual effort to restore a healthy, natural order and to displace an unhealthy social order. His concern over bread embodied this struggle: In the 1840s Graham accused commercial bakers of using poor flour and adulterating their breads with "bean flour, peas and potatoes, chalk, pipe clay, and plaster of Paris."[15] Like many health reformers of the time, Graham thought that people should avoid refined-flour bread and consume whole-grain bread baked at home by the wife and mother of each household. By centering this important part of the family's food procurement at home, he aimed to fend off the unnatural social order brought about by commercialization.

Physician William Andrus Alcott (1798–1859), a contemporary of Graham's, also promoted vegetarianism as a way to avoid excessive stimulation. He was influenced especially by his cousin, transcendentalist Amos Bronson Alcott, father of author Louisa May Alcott and founder of the vegan commune Fruitlands. William Alcott received his medical and surgical license from Yale University in 1825, after attending a five-month series of lectures there, and he published over a hundred books on health, diet, and ethics in his lifetime, including many books that gave advice to young people.[16] He argued against using manure (as a form of forced fertilization), producing food in greenhouses (as a form of forced vegetation), and consuming decaying fruits and vegetables. He promoted the idea that "diseased food causes disease in people who use it,"[17] and he considered meat to be the most "unnatural" food.

In 1851, Alcott wrote that "vegetable diet lies at the basis of all reform, whether civil, social, moral, or religious."[18] The vegetarian diet (also called the natural diet and Pythagorean diet) was an integral part of other reform movements in the Jacksonian period—including temperance, suffrage, women's dress reform, and abolition—and many feminist and abolitionist leaders, such as Susan B. Anthony, Lucy Stone, Amelia Bloomer, and Horace Greeley, attended early meetings of the American Vegetarian Society, which had been founded in 1850 by William Metcalfe, Sylvester Graham, William Alcott, Russell Trall, and others.[19]

Also in the mid-1800s, a group of religious sectarians began the Seventh Day Adventist Church as a reaction to the inaccurate Millerite prophecy that the world would end on

October 22, 1844. Inspired by one of its leaders, Ellen White, this new religion advocated a vegetarian diet as a healthful way to better serve God. In 1855, religious leaders established their headquarters in Battle Creek, Michigan. There they also established the Western Health Reform Institute, later known as the Battle Creek Sanatorium, where John Harvey Kellogg (1852–1945)—originator of granola and cornflakes, who had earned his medical degree from Bellevue Medical College in New York—continued Graham's legacy from the 1870s into the twentieth century.[20]

Seventh Day Adventists have historically and contemporarily played an important role in the spread of vegetarian principles and information.[21] Although the religion does not mandate vegetarianism, today about one-half of the estimated five hundred thousand U. S. Seventh Day Adventists follow a vegetarian diet, and most of the rest consume comparatively less meat than does the general population.[22] The fact that church members constitute a large, definable, vegetarian population enables researchers to conduct longitudinal studies on the health consequences of following a vegetarian diet.[23] The Seventh Day Adventist church has contributed significantly to the spread of vegetarian ideas and knowledge through the establishment of a research institution, Loma Linda University (which has published its research data in mainstream and medical and nutritional journals since the 1950s);[24] a health foods corporation, Worthington Foods; a chain of restaurants, Country Life; and a magazine, *Vibrant Life*.

This brief historical overview suggests that the vegetarian movement in North America has consistently focused on health issues. The early vegetarian movement certainly had the spiritual component of viewing vegetarianism as an opportunity for individuals to align themselves with the Divine and to strive for personal improvement. With the rise of positivist science in the nineteenth century, however, advocates needed to focus on demonstrating the health benefits—or at the very least, the lack of health risks—associated with vegetarian diets, a concern that persists even today.

The Health Professions' Approaches to Vegetarian Diets

Nineteenth-century advocates of conventional, or "regular," medicine disparaged their vegetarian, or "irregular," counterparts. Seeking to legitimize their own practices, conventional practitioners in the mid-1800s established the American Medical Association (AMA), labeling most of their less-conventional counterparts as "quacks."[25] Vegetarians were the subject of much popular humor, as "fun was poked at the vegetarians on the printed page, in comic opera and in newspapers."[26] According to historian James Whorton, the regulars "had much merriment at vegetarians' expense," characterizing vegetarian women as "mummies preserved in saffron" and vegetarian men as "lean-visaged cadaverous disciples" of Graham."[27] Vegetarians were often portrayed in popular culture as sallow, wan, and emaciated.

In the twentieth century, nutritional scientists have paid significant attention to not only the health consequences but also some of the social aspects of vegetarian diets. In the 1970s—in the *Journal of the American Dietetic Association, Nutrition Today,* and other research journals—nutritional scientists began to use the term "new vegetarians" to indicate converts to vegetarianism as distinguished from those who grew up following vegetarian diets as part of a religious doctrine (for example, the Seventh Day Adventists, the Hindus, or the Jains). Johanna T. Dwyer and Jean Mayer characterized many of these "new vegetarians" as former "hard drug" users who had adopted vegetarian diets as "a crutch which helps them to refrain from relapsing into drug use."[28] In some of the nutritional science literature of the 1970s, writers used "new vegetarian" interchangeably with two derogatory terms that nutritional scientists had commonly used previously to describe vegetarians: "food cultist" and "food faddist."[29]

In the 1970s, many nutritionists characterized vegetarian diets as medically unsound. A substantial amount of research focused on the problem of underweight vegetarian children, and some researchers called the feeding of vegan diets to children a form of child abuse.[30] A section of Darla Erhard's 1973 article in *Nutrition Today*, for example, bears the subtitle "A Starved Child of the New Vegetarians." The opening paragraph reads as follows: "Recently an infant was admitted to the San Francisco General Hospital representing all the problems one faces in dealing with the children of the new vegetarians. There was the deplorable condition of the child itself, the difficulty of convincing a reluctant mother of the staff's benevolent intentions and the downright opposition of an elusive father. It's an instructive case history."[31] Later the author reveals that the parents belonged to "the Vegan Society, a cult of rigid dietary concepts."[32] In a 1974 article, Erhard presents a "wheel of vegetarianism" representing various approaches to vegetarian eating; at the center of the wheel, she inscribes "unscientific vegetarianism" and "food faddism."[33] Although the author concedes that vegetarian diets and food "cults . . . have contributed to the health and peace of mind of a great many young people," she warns that these diets provide adequate nutrition only when they include dairy and poultry products.[34]

Although most medical research reports since the 1980s have focused on the adequacies rather than the inadequacies of vegetarian diets,[35] Erhard's portrayal of vegetarianism as potentially hazardous has persisted with respect to certain segments of the population: young children and teenage girls, in particular. In several recent cases, parents have been charged with neglect and have lost custody of their children, at least in part for feeding them vegetarian diets.[36] As this chapter discusses later in more detail, even stronger concerns have emerged over the suggestion that children do not need and in fact should not drink milk. And some psychologists have viewed young women's adherence to vegetarian diets as a possible "warning sign" for a masked eating disorder.[37] Other psychologists have suggested that many young women adopt a vegetarian or partially vegetarian diet *after* the onset of anorexia nervosa. Nevertheless, linking vegetarian diets to undesirable thinness and to possible psychological problems can evoke public concern, especially among parents of adolescent girls.[38] Except perhaps for young children and adolescent females prone to anorexia, since the 1980s, vegetarian diets have experienced increased public acceptance and have become increasingly available in public programs such as school lunches. This has been spurred, in large part, by approval from mainstream physicians and from such organizations as the ADA and the USDA.

Vegetarian Diets and the ADA

In 1980, the ADA began to issue periodic position papers on vegetarian diets.[39] The position papers go through an ADA peer-review process, after which the ADA House of Delegates votes for approval or revision. Consistently, the ADA position papers have supported vegetarian and vegan diets as dietary options. Despite the cautious tone of the ADA's original 1980 position paper—which provides background information about vegetarians and vegetarian diets, including an extensive "definition of terms" section and heavy reliance on the Seventh Day Adventist studies—it effectively dispelled the idea that all vegetarian diets were faddist and harmful.

Subsequent editions of the position paper have taken an increasingly positive stance on vegetarian diets. The 1997 position paper states, "Scientific data suggest positive relationships between a vegetarian diet and reduced risk for several chronic degenerative diseases and conditions, including obesity, coronary artery disease, hypertension, diabetes mellitus, and some types of cancer. Vegetarian diets, like all diets, need to be planned appropriately to be nutritionally adequate."[40] The position papers also give substantial consideration to how to plan healthful vegetarian diets—with or without dairy products. The 1997 position paper, for example, introduces the Food Guide Pyramid for Vegetarian Meal Planning. This is a version of the USDA food pyramid, which grounds a vegetarian diet on the "bread, cereal, rice, and pasta group," followed by a "vegetable group" and "fruit group," a "dry beans, nuts, seeds, eggs, and meat-substitutes group," an optional "milk, yogurt, and cheese group," and a "use sparingly" "fats, oils, and sweets" group.[41]

In addition, the ADA sponsors a Dietetic Practice Group with over seventeen hundred members, which "serves as a link in providing accurate information, resources, and support for those who promote sound nutrition based primarily or exclusively on plant foods."[42] The ADA also publishes and distributes the brochure "Eating Well—the Vegetarian Way," which not only defines the different types of vegetarian diets, evaluates their nutritional adequacy, and provides vegetarian menu suggestions but also reads like a public presentation of the 1997 ADA position paper. The 1992 brochure lists several health benefits, stating that "heart disease, high blood pressure, adult-onset diabetes, obesity, and some forms of cancer tend to develop less often in vegetarians than in non-vegetarians." Other than vitamin-B_{12} supplementation for vegans and vitamin-D supplementation for vegetarians and vegans who do not consume dairy products and who are not directly exposed to natural sunlight on a regular basis, the brochure includes no cautions regarding the ability of vegetarian diets to meet nutritional requirements.

Vegetarian Diets and the USDA

Unlike the ADA, the U.S. government only recently acknowledged the adequacy of vegetarian diets. In the 1995

U.S. Government Dietary Recommendations, for the first time, the Department of Health and Human Services and the USDA referred to vegetarian diets as acceptable options: "Some Americans eat vegetarian diets for reasons of culture, belief, or health. Most vegetarians eat milk products and eggs, and as a group, these lacto-ovo-vegetarians enjoy excellent health. Vegetarian diets are consistent with the *Dietary Guidelines for Americans* and can meet Recommended Dietary Allowances for nutrients."[43] This first-time inclusion initiated a spate of questions at the White House press conference announcing the release of the recommendations. On January 2, 1996, C-Span broadcast the following exchange: To the question "What kind of reaction [have you] received to the nod toward a vegetarian diet from an important constituent of agriculture—the cattlemen, the poultry producers, and the producers of the 'other white meat?'" Agriculture Secretary Dan Glickman responded:

> What we have said here is that if you have a vegetarian diet you *can* get your nutrients, if it's carefully balanced. But we also point out quite clearly in the Food Pyramid that a balanced diet includes meats and fish and chicken, and that's an important part of a balanced diet. . . . If an individual wants to go down the vegetarian route, he or she can get their nutrients that way, but they have to be a lot more careful and a lot more creative, and a lot more imaginative to make sure their nutrients are in that kind of balance.

Glickman's response suggests USDA *acceptance*, rather than outright *endorsement*, of vegetarian diets.

Vegetarian Diets and Physicians

Physicians have been slower to legitimize vegetarian diets than have dietitians. Although physicians recognize the importance of diet in the etiology of conditions such as heart disease and cancer, they do not necessarily recognize vegetarian diets as either preventive or palliative. For example, Dr. Neil Barnard, director of PCRM, and two colleagues published a peer-reviewed journal article in *Preventive Medicine* (using secondary research) that estimated that meat eating directly caused between $28.6 billion and $61.4 billion in medical care costs for 1992. However, a spokesperson for the AMA disputed their claims, stating that Barnard and his colleagues had neglected to control adequately for other factors, such as age, sex, and genetic history.[44]

In general, conventional medical practitioners pay little attention to diet, and they rarely provide nutrition education to their patients. Many physicians have received little or no nutritional training themselves; in 1993 only about 25 percent of medical schools required their students to take nutrition courses. Less than 60 percent of physicians report that they have received nutritional training, and many cite barriers—such as lack of time, patient compliance, and knowledge of nutrition—to the practice of providing patients with nutritional consultations.[45]

Recently, however, physicians have begun to pay more attention to alternative treatments, some of which include shifts toward more plant-based diets. One point of interest is the work of physician Dean Ornish, director of the Preventive Medicine Research Institute at the University of California at San Francisco since 1970. Ornish's program, which was first publicly outlined in *Stress, Diet and Your Heart* in 1982, has explored alternative ways of combating heart disease, including the use of stress reduction and radical dietary change as methods of reversing severe arterial sclerosis.[46] The program includes a near-vegan diet, which nets a daily fat intake of less than 10 percent, as well as a daily exercise and relaxation regimen. In an early controlled experiment, Ornish's clients experienced a 50-percent increase in blood flow to the heart and a 40-percent drop in their cholesterol level; the control group's condition worsened slightly during the same period.[47] Other longitudinal controlled trial studies, published in the *Journal of the American Medical Association*, document the reduction of arterial heart abnormalities in those who follow the Ornish program.[48]

Ornish, who served as a nutritional advisor to the Clinton White House, offers a week-long residential program four times a year at a retreat center in California. Other such programs, modeled on Ornish's, have been offered at large hospitals such as the Beth Israel Hospitals in New York and Boston and Richland Hospital in Columbia, South Carolina. Health insurance companies, such as Blue Cross/Blue Shield and Mutual of Omaha, are beginning to offer compensation for the thirty-six-hundred-dollar cost of the week-long program, hoping to reduce the number of fifty-thousand-dollar coronary by-pass operations.[49] Although Ornish's research has been validated and accepted, the medical community seems to doubt the public's capacity to make major dietary changes, even in a health crisis. According to Dr. Eugene Brunwald of the Harvard Medical School, "It's a valuable demonstration that when you go all-out and pull out all the stops, that lifestyle changes can reverse athero sclerosis, coronary artery disease. . . . There are very, very few people who will be prepared to make that lifestyle change, and there will be few people who will be prepared to motivate them, as Dr. Ornish did so successfully."[50] Although Ornish has conducted his research and published his results within the domain of conventional medicine, his program has often been dismissed as impractical. As more longitudinal data regarding program participants become available and more health insurance companies opt to cover the costs of the program, however, this pattern is likely to change.

Two Controversies: Confronting Concerns about Protein and Calcium

The 1990s witnessed a growing scientific acceptance of well-planned ovo-lacto-vegetarian diets. Where concerns remain about the risks of these diets to the health of children and adolescent females, suggestions are offered about how to improve vegetarian diets for these populations. The acceptance of ovo-lacto-vegetarian diets is strongly supported by extensive research that shows that healthful and varied versions of these diets can easily provide all of the Recommended Daily Allowances for nutrients—including protein. For many years, as we discuss in more detail later, public reservations about the healthfulness of ovo-lacto-vegetarian diets centered on the belief that plant protein was inferior to meat protein and that these "low-quality" protein foods needed to be carefully combined in order to achieve protein comparable to that in meat. Although vegetarians still frequently encounter the question "Where do you get your protein?" they can now supply answers supported by the legitimacy of such organizations as the ADA and the USDA. Overcoming the "protein-complementarity myth" has made it much easier to promote ovo-lacto-vegetarianism on health grounds.

As the myth slowly fades, a new controversy takes its place—a controversy that is key to the public acceptance of veganism. Whereas meat has long been associated with strength and vigor, milk has an even more sacred connection: It is associated with purity, balance, innocence and with strong bones and teeth and a healthy complexion. Overriding milk's positive associations may be even more difficult to accomplish than was erasing the protein-complementarity myth.

A Slowly Fading Controversy: Is Meat Protein Better Than Vegetable Protein?

In the 1960s and 1970s, a hippie counterculture that moved people to consider the political implications of their food choices and to return to a more natural lifestyle played a large part in increasing public interest in vegetarian diets.[51] Much of the concern that nutritionists and dietitians expressed about countercultural "new vegetarians" focused on protein, a nutrient strongly associated with strength, vigor, and meat. In the 1970s, a persistent notion about the inferiority of plant protein made vegetarianism seem like a difficult, risky, and somewhat unnatural practice.

A key influential book, Lappé's 1971 *Diet for a Small Planet*, however, moved many people to adopt vegetarian or semivegetarian diets. Lappé's idea was that if the massive resources associated with animal food production were used for plant cultivation, many more people could be fed. A down-to-earth, straightforward, and seemingly well-researched text, *Diet for a Small Planet* "promised personal adventure, growth, and liberation through culinary adventure."[52] The book, which sold almost two million copies in ten years, provided not only an ecological argument for vegetarianism but also a collection of vegetarian recipes and an explanation of vegetable protein.

Lappé told readers that, by combining certain foods, they could get as much as or more than the amount of "high-quality" protein that they could get from meat:

> Obviously the best solution is to . . . [combine] different plant sources, or nonmeat animal protein sources with plant sources, in the *same* meal. Most people do this to some extent anyway, just as a matter of course. Eating a mixture of protein sources can increase the protein value of the meal; here's a case where *the whole is greater than the sum of its parts.* . . . Eating wheat and protein together, for example, can increase by about 33 percent the protein actually usable by your body. . . . To exploit this complementarity effect, you can make dishes and plan meals so that the protein in one food fills the amino acid deficiencies in another food.[53]

Lappé's approach, which suggested that protein combining was fairly complicated, included numerous tables that charted how the proteins in various foods could complement one another. Her intention was to show that a vegetarian diet could be healthful, interesting, and helpful to the environment. Instead, however, Lappé inadvertently reinforced the ideas that plant protein was lower quality than meat protein; that vegetarians needed to give careful thought to protein in their meal planning; and that, without careful planning, vegetarian diets constituted a health risk.

At about the same time, scientific and professional organizations reinforced the notion that vegetarian diets must include complementary proteins. The National Research Council, for example, released this statement in 1974:

> The quality of proteins in plant foods, notably cereal grains, is generally lower than that of animal proteins. Protein quality is dependent on the amounts and the utilization of eight of the twenty constituent amino acids in protein. Protein foods of animal origin contain these eight amino acids in nearly optimum amounts and in an available form, and thus are said to be high-quality proteins. On the other hand, cereal grain proteins are relatively low in the essential amino acid lysine, and thus provide lower-quality protein. Legumes, such as dried beans and peas, contain ample lysine, but are relatively low in methionine, so they also provide protein of marginal quality. When the cereal and legume proteins are eaten together, the methionine provided by the cereal grain and the lysine provided by the legume improve the "balance" in the amino acid supply and the mixture of proteins is of better quality than that provided by either alone.[54]

Similarly, the ADA included the following statement in its 1975 "Position Paper on Food and Nutrition Misinformation on Selected Topics":

> The American Dietetic Association recognizes the quality of vegetable protein is less than animal protein, but the careful selection of foods for vegetarian diets can insure adequate nutrition for adults. Combinations of legumes, grains, seeds, and nuts (beans with corn, beans with rice, or peanuts with wheat) can provide adequate dietary protein for adults. Infants and children two to five years of age need more protein for growth and devel-

opment than is likely to be available from pure vegetarian [vegan] diets.[55]

Although such scientific observations gave Lappé's work credibility, they also strengthened the idea that there was cause for vegetarians to worry about their diets.

The 1980s brought an increased acceptance of vegetarian diets among health professionals, but the notion of protein complementarity persisted. Although the ADA's first "Position Paper on the Vegetarian Approach to Eating," published in 1980, discussed vegetarian diets in a more positive tone than had much of the 1970s scientific literature, it promoted the idea of complementary proteins:

> Although plant foods have a lower coefficient of digestibility and their essential amino acid patterns are usually not as well balanced as in animal sources, a *mixture* of proteins from largely unrefined grains, legumes, seeds, nuts, and vegetables—especially dark green, leafy vegetables—supplement each other so that all the essential amino acids are available in sufficient quantity. . . . Combinations of grains and legumes, the principal sources of protein for total vegetarians, are good examples of complementation occurring naturally among plant foods.[56]

Then, in 1988, while preparing to co-draft (with Dwyer) an updated ADA position paper on vegetarian diets, Suzanne Havala questioned the necessity of complementing proteins. As Havala later explained:

> There was no basis for that that I could see. And at that point, nobody was saying that you didn't have to complement proteins. That was something I didn't understand, and it didn't make any sense to me. And I began calling around and talking to people and asking them what the justification was for saying that you had to complement proteins, and there was none. And what I got instead was some interesting insight from people who were knowledgeable and actually felt that there was probably no need to complement proteins. So we went ahead and made that change in the paper. And it was a couple of years after that that

Vernon Young and Peter Pellet published their paper that became the definitive contemporary guide to protein metabolism in humans. And it also confirmed that complementing proteins at meals was totally unnecessary.[57]

The 1988 ADA position paper, approved by peer review and by a delegation vote, provided a revised view of protein in vegetarian diets: "Mixtures of proteins from grains, vegetables, legumes, seeds, and nuts eaten over the course of the day complement one another in their amino acid profiles without the necessity of precise planning and complementation of proteins within each meal, as the recently popular 'combined proteins theory' has urged."[58]

Today the official position of both the USDA and the ADA is that vegetarians whose diets are generally healthful do not need to worry about complementing proteins. According to the U.S. Dietary Guidelines, "You can get enough protein from a vegetarian diet as long as the variety and amounts of foods consumed are adequate."[59] The ADA's "Eating Well—The Vegetarian Way" brochure states that "vegetarians do not need to combine specific foods within a meal as the old 'complementary protein' theory advised. The body makes its own complete proteins if a variety of plant foods—fruits, vegetables, grains, legumes, nuts, and seeds—and enough calories are eaten during the day."[60] By the mid-1990s, it seemed that, as long as their diets were varied, healthful, and included enough calories, there was no reason to question vegetarians' protein consumption.

Although the protein-complementarity myth has faded somewhat since the publication of *Diet for a Small Planet,* many cookbooks and professional publications still promote the idea today. For example, the Dietitians for Canada fact sheet, "Celebrating the Pleasure of Vegetarian Eating," states, "If you do not include any animal products in your diet, combining grains with legumes, nuts and seeds, and vegetables daily will provide tasty meals and help you meet your protein

needs." The fact sheet then goes on to offer suggestions including the following: "Peanut Butter Sandwich, Lentil Soup
with Crackers, . . . Red Beans and Rice, [and] Bean Salad with
Whole-Grain Cereal topping."[61] Similarly, the American Academy of Pediatrics 1999 *Guide to Your Child's Nutrition*
states:

> People on vegetarian diets take care of their protein needs by
> pairing plant foods that balance each other's shortfalls. Pairing
> foods in this way is called protein complementation. Eating a
> grain and a legume does the trick; beans and tortillas, a peanut
> butter sandwich on wheat bread, and black-eyed peas and rice
> are good examples of protein complementation. You can also
> compensate for any lack in a plant-based food by adding a small
> amount of animal protein, such as in pasta with cheese or cereal
> with milk.[62]

These menu suggestions all reinforce the idea that to follow a
vegetarian diet that does not include these particular combi-
nations (and especially a diet that does not include eggs or
milk) is a health risk.

A Current Controversy: Milk—Does It Do a Body Good?

Today, many people view an ovo-lacto-vegetarian diet as potentially very healthful and a semivegetarian diet as optimal; in
one study, one-third of adults said that "their diets would be
healthier if they did not eat red meat."[63] Although some concern about the potential protein inadequacies of vegetarian
diets still exists (for example, for some athletes and for people
who follow protein-centered diets such as "The Zone"),[64]
and some professional organizations still advocate protein
complementarity, protein in vegetarian diets has become less
of an issue over time.

In contrast, most people consider dairy products to be important—perhaps even indispensable—to a healthful diet.

"Milk . . . stands as a restorative, a symbol of purity, the innocence of a child, natural goodness, calm strength and reality."[65] Recent concern about the high fat content of dairy foods has been put to rest with the advent of new low-fat and nonfat dairy products, and the majority of consumers perceive yogurt to be an "exceptionally healthy food."[66]

In a Wisconsin Dairy Council news release, Robert Heaney, a professor of medicine at Creighton University, states, "Milk is an essential part of any diet. The adverse consequences of eliminating dairy products from one's diet are enormous."[67] For most people, milk is a primary source of calcium; however, many other foods provide this nutrient. The ADA's 1997 position paper on vegetarian diets—which includes an extensive list of legumes (such as chickpeas and black beans), soyfoods (such as tofu and fortified soy milk), and vegetables (such as broccoli and collard greens)—states that vegetarians can easily get all of their calcium requirements from plant-based sources.[68] The USDA's Dietary Guidelines for Americans lists several "good sources of calcium," including dark-green leafy vegetables, tofu, and tortillas made from lime-processed corn.[69]

Even though many foods provide high levels of calcium, most nutrition and medical professionals hold that consumption of low-fat or nonfat dairy products is the best—or at least the easiest—way to meet Recommended Daily Allowances. "Does anyone seriously think that the general public is going to drink soymilk?" asks Jeanne Goldberg, director of the Center on Nutrition Communication at Tufts University.[70] According to "Healthy People 2000," a 1991 U.S. Department of Health and Human Services report, "With current food selection practices in the United States, use of dairy products constitutes the difference between inadequate and adequate intakes of calcium." If people were to stop eating dairy products, worry nutritional scientists and dietitians, their already marginal intake levels of calcium might drop.

Special concern is focused on the elimination of dairy foods from children's diets. Despite the ADA's position that calcium and vitamin-D deficiencies are unlikely in children whose diets are well planned,[71] many physicians and nutritionists still regard vegetarian (and especially vegan) diets as dangerous. The 1998 edition of *Dr. Spock's Baby and Child Care* created a stir, for example, by suggesting that ideally parents should provide a vegan diet for their children after age two: "We used to think of cow's milk as a nearly perfect food. However, over the past several years, researchers have found new information that has caused many of us to change our opinion. This has provoked a lot of understandable controversy, but I have come to believe that cow's milk is not necessary for children."[72] In response, pediatrician T. Berry Brazelton "called his new dietary recommendations 'absolutely insane. . . . A vegetarian diet doesn't make any sense. Meat is an excellent source of the iron and protein children need, and to take milk away from children—I think that's really dangerous. Milk is needed for calcium and vitamin D.'"[73] The American Academy of Pediatrics *Guide to Your Child's Nutrition* lists additional concerns: "Children who are fed the vegan diet suggested by Dr. Spock must have supplements or fortified foods to replace essential nutrients that are missing in a vegetarian diet."[74] The book identifies several "problem areas," including adequate calories, protein, vitamin B_{12}, vitamin D, calcium, and zinc. Reactions such as these strongly reinforce the idea that milk is essential to good health, especially for children.

The emerging controversy about dairy products centers on two related questions: (1) Do people *need* dairy products for good health? (2) Are dairy products healthful or unhealthful? The ADA, the USDA, and other groups lend support to campaigns for vegan diets by stating that dairy products are not necessary for good health. However, the American Academy of Pediatrics, Health Canada, and other groups promote the importance of dairy products for children. Much less support exists for the argument that dairy products are harmful and should be minimized in or eliminated from people's diets. People often think of milk, and especially yogurt, as health foods. Advertising campaigns such as "Milk—It Does a Body Good" and "Got Milk?" reinforce the belief that drinking milk is the best way to build strong bones and to prevent the development of osteoporosis. The milk mustache campaign sponsored by the National Fluid Milk Processor Promotion Board, with a 1998 budget of $190 million, used well-known and respected actors, athletes, and government officials to attack public perceptions that milk is a high-fat product good for kids only.[75]

Those who have tried to counter the notion that milk is healthful have met with minimal success. For example, since the early 1990s, PCRM has charged that dairy foods cause a wide variety of health problems and that milk often contains potentially dangerous contaminants.[76] In the late 1990s, PCRM appeared to switch its campaign strategy from its focus on the negative qualities of dairy products. In 1999, PCRM initiated a campaign countering the notion that dairy products are needed to help protect against bone fractures and osteoporosis and suggesting that plant-based diets supply adequate calcium more healthfully. In addition, PCRM filed a petition with the Federal Trade Commission against the National Fluid Milk Processor Promotion Board's milk mustache advertisements, claiming that they mislead consumers about the health benefits of milk. PCRM's petition cites studies that suggest that female milk drinkers suffer as many fractures as or more fractures than women who avoid milk. PCRM also claims that the advertisements—which feature such celebrities as Vanessa Williams, Spike Lee, and Whoopi Goldberg—suggest inaccurate health benefits for African Americans, who have not been shown to benefit from increased calcium intake.[77]

The dairy industry and some health organizations dismiss PCRM's efforts as biased and unscientific. For example, an American Council on Science and Health publication about "the milk controversy" states:

> The Physicians' Committee for Responsible Medicine may have been motivated to overstate its case against cows' milk because it has another agenda. The organization strongly supports total vegetarianism. . . . PCRM also opposes the use of animals in medical research and education, and it offers for sale a variety of publications that strongly support the concept of animal rights. It is possible that these views may have influenced PCRM's judgment on the health effects of cows' milk.[78]

Similarly, a Milk Industry Federation spokesperson calls PCRM's new campaign "irresponsible" and an "incorrect reading of the science."[79] Considering people's generally positive view of dairy foods and the dairy industry's immense resources, it would seem that—barring a diary foods contamination crisis—little is likely to convince the general public that it would be beneficial to their health to switch to plant-food sources of calcium.

Implications of Health Controversies for the Vegetarian Movement

Historically, North American vegetarianism, grounded in the ideas and practices of Jacksonian reformers, has focused on diet as a means of self-improvement and self-transformation. Today, most people who adopt vegetarianism expect to become healthier as they gradually eliminate animal products from their diets. Approval from mainstream health practitioners and organizations, such as the ADA and the USDA, helps promote vegetarianism on health grounds.

To date, however, no mainstream health organization has questioned the health value of dairy products. Although the ADA and the USDA recommend the reduction of fat in our diets and list a variety of plant-based sources of calcium, lingering concerns about the necessity or desirability of dairy products (especially for children and pregnant women) hinder the promotion of veganism over ovo-lacto- or lacto-vegetarianism.

As the dairy and meat industries develop and market lower-fat, lower-calorie products, many people who have reduced or eliminated their consumption of animal products are likely to start eating them again. Although health interests may move people toward vegetarianism, without commitment to a vegetarian identity, the convenience of a meat-based diet has a good chance of pulling them back. Thus, promoting concern for animals and the environment is essential to the advancement of the vegetarian movement. Health-motivated semivegetarians help the movement peripherally, by demanding more vegetarian products and by making vegetarianism more socially acceptable, but they rarely contribute resources to the movement directly. At present, although PCRM has made a concerted effort to do so, no vegetarian-oriented organization has the power to overcome meat and dairy interests. The number of committed, strongly motivated advocates must increase significantly if the movement is to confront these major industries in any meaningful way.

Many vegetarian organizations find themselves in the difficult position of wanting to promote the ethical reasons for adopting veganism without alienating their health-motivated ovo-lacto-vegetarians. Because most people become vegetarians gradually and many even initially increase their egg and dairy consumption to compensate for the meat that they have eliminated from their diets, strong vegan messages may scare away potential adherents. Later chapters explore how vegetarian organizations have tried to negotiate this challenge.

Clearly, the gradual validation of vegetarian diets by mainstream health and government organizations has contributed to their social acceptance. Vegetarian organizations frequently support the health benefits of vegetarianism by citing documents such as the ADA's position papers on vegetarian diets and the USDA's Dietary Recommendations for Americans. Periodicals such as *Vegetarian Times, Vegetarian Journal,* and *Vegetarian Voice* include articles written by and about physicians and registered dietitians who review current nutritional and medical research and who advocate vegetarianism. Confirming the health benefits of vegetarian diets is key to winning new adherents.

3 Charting the Contemporary Vegetarian Movement in the Social Movement Field

We as a movement need to identify and find ways to support struggling groups, as well as help medium-size groups become larger and larger. *It is our goal to establish viable and expanding vegetarian groups in every metropolitan area of North America.* If we can do this, we will be able to present our case to the public in North America and throughout the world.

—Vegetarian Union of North America, "Guide for Local Vegetarian Groups"

Social movement activity is much more complex than it seems at first glance. When we think of a social movement, we might think of a single entity consistently acting as a unit. In reality, however, a movement comprises many parts that may or may not work together as a functioning whole. At the same time, a social movement does not exist in isolation; it depends on reactions from other movements and countermovements in the social movement field. Related movements can provide alliances and bases for potential new members. By provoking controversy and bringing attention to goals and ideas, countermovements can also benefit a social movement.

Since the 1960s, social scientists have increasingly addressed social movements that focus on transforming individ-

47

uals and cultural beliefs. Often identifying these movements as new, they suggest that they differ in some way from the old political movements that aimed to topple power structures and transform economic relations by changing the structural arrangements of society. Whereas political movements attempt to shift the structured imbalance of power and resources within a social system, cultural movements work to generate collective social identities, motivate personal transformation, and manipulate common beliefs and ideas.[1] Cultural movements use cultural products such as values, beliefs, stories, art, and literature to spur collective change. Although adversarial conflict may be less visible in a cultural than in a political movement, cultural movements often engage in symbolic conflict with the dominant culture.[2]

The vegetarian movement in particular typically makes a concerted effort to minimize conflict. Although movement advocates occasionally battle meat producers and meat eaters, they primarily counter the cultural notion that animals should be used as human food. The movement as a whole attempts to create a culture that is more tolerant of vegetarianism as it simultaneously moves individuals in the same direction. Vegetarian organizations are central to these goals.

Boundaries of the Contemporary Vegetarian Movement

Although many organizations in some way promote vegetarianism, few openly identify as vegetarian organizations designed primarily to promote the vegetarian movement. Taken together, however, the many groups and individuals that support vegetarian principles constitute a much broader vegetarian movement than the relatively small number of explicitly vegetarian organizations suggests. National animal rights groups, such as People for the Ethical Treatment of Animals (PETA), Last Chance for Animals (LCA), and Animal Rights International (ARI), actively promote veganism. And many writers and speakers, including health care professionals who support vegetarianism, contribute to movement activity.

The vegetarian movement includes all activities and ideas that center on promoting vegetarian and vegan diets:

- *Political Change Activities:* efforts to make concrete changes through governmental actions that help promote vegetarian diets (for example, working to change federal School Lunch Program requirements to accommodate a nutrient-based standard that does not require meat)
- *Cultural Change Activities:* efforts to make the culture more vegetarian friendly (for example, encouraging restaurants to offer vegetarian entrées)
- *Personal Change Activities:* efforts to encourage people to adopt vegetarianism (for example, sponsoring vegetarian potluck dinners and food-tasting events and distributing educational materials)

Many and varied individuals and groups support vegetarian organizations in carrying out these activities, which are central to the movement's promotion of personal, cultural, and social change.

A Basic Chronology of Contemporary Vegetarian Movement Organizations

The North American vegetarian movement includes both national and local organizations, all of which except for VRG— now a national organization—have maintained their geographic scope over time. Membership in vegetarian organizations is small compared with membership in animal rights groups. For example, whereas PETA had 300,000 paying members in 1995; Farm Sanctuary had 35,000, VRG had 16,500, and the North American Vegetarian Society (NAVS) had about 4,000.[3]

Because many groups engage in similar kinds of activities, it is not easy to categorize national vegetarian organizations.

Some groups provide information primarily to their affiliates and to the general public, whereas others are directly involved with institutional change as well. Still others adopt more of a direct-action approach, encouraging individuals and groups of activists to engage in activities that challenge the general public's attitudes about meat (see Table 3). All of these groups . encourage people to effect personal change first and to adopt a nonviolent, open-minded approach to changing others.

Public Outreach/Educational Organizations

The American Vegan Society (AVS), NAVS, and the Vegetarian Union of North America (VUNA) all focus on providing educational materials to prospective members and educating current vegetarians through organizational publications and conferences.

The 1960 founding of AVS marks the beginning of the contemporary vegetarian movement in North America. Although some local vegetarian organizations have been in existence since before 1960—such as the Vegetarian Society of Washington, D.C. (circa 1927), and the Toronto Vegetarian Association (circa 1945)—AVS is the first contemporary national organization. Its founding marks the beginning of intensified vegetarian activity at both local and national levels.

Table 3   National Vegetarian Organizations

Type	Organization
Public outreach/ education	American Vegan Society (AVS) North American Vegetarian Society (NAVS) Vegetarian Union of North America (VUNA)
Institutional change/ education	EarthSave International Vegetarian Resource Group (VRG) Farm Sanctuary
Grassroots activist/ education	FARM Vegan Outreach Vegan Action

Shortly after becoming a vegan in the late 1950s, lifelong vegetarian H. Jay Dinshah (1933–2000) founded AVS. Throughout the 1960s, AVS served as both a vegetarian and a vegan organization. Its focus was primarily outreach through such publications as *Ahimsa,* the group's magazine; *Here's Harmlessness,* a collection of vegan testimonials; and *Out of the Jungle,* a book on veganism and nonviolence.[4]

AVS later created two other national groups, NAVS and VUNA. In 1973, Dinshah and some of his American colleagues attended a World Vegetarian Congress in Sweden. When they offered to hold the next World Vegetarian Congress in the United States, they were told that, in order to do so, they would have to establish a national *vegetarian* organization separate from the national *vegan* group. Thus, NAVS, which shared office space and personnel with AVS for several years, was born.

In the late 1970s, NAVS moved to its own office in Dolgeville, New York, and in 1975, the organization published its first issue of *Vegetarian Voice,* a magazine that primarily addresses health and dietary issues. Since that time, NAVS has published and distributed a number of booklets, including "Vegetarianism: Tipping the Scales for the Environment," "Vegetarianism: Answers to the Most Commonly Asked Questions," and "The Care and Feeding of Vegetarians: A 'How-To' Guide for Non-Vegetarians." NAVS also originated the annual celebration of World Vegetarian Day and sponsors the Vegetarian Express Fast Food Campaign, encouraging people to call for fast-food chains to serve more vegetarian foods.

VUNA was founded by AVS to represent North America in the International Vegetarian Union (IVU), a primarily symbolic organization founded in 1908 that hosts the biennial World Vegetarian Congress. VUNA is a "network of vegetarian groups throughout the U.S. and Canada,"[5] which, unlike NAVS, has neither paid employees nor a central office. In 1995, VUNA published the booklet "Guide for Local Vegetarian Groups: How to Start, Maintain, and Expand Your Local Vegetarian Group," which includes information on how to attract volunteers, incorporate as a nonprofit organization, and sponsor group activities. Large local vegetarian societies in Toronto, Boston, Louisville, and Seattle have sponsored festivals that celebrate vegetarian foods and ideas and generate media publicity. VUNA is currently working on a publication entitled "Vegetarian Food Fair Manual," intended to help smaller groups organize similar events.[6]

Institutional Change/Educational Organizations

The organizations EarthSave International, VRG, and Farm Sanctuary combine their efforts to educate the public with efforts to effect change in cultural and social institutions.

After intended heir to the Baskin Robbins ice cream fortune John Robbins rejected his family's lifestyle and authored the 1987 book *Diet for a New America*,[7] he set about to found a group devoted to both education and institutional change. Originally called Concerned Citizens for Planet Earth, Robbins's organization, EarthSave International, focuses on the effects of food choices on the environment. EarthSave International advocates typically avoid the terms "vegan" and "vegetarian" diets, choosing instead to promote "plant-based" diets in an effort to bridge the gap between meat eaters and vegetarians. Stacey Vicari explains the concept: "Meat-based doesn't mean that all you eat is meat. . . . The bulk of your diet is animal products. Plant-based means that the bulk of your diet is going to [comprise] plant-based foods. . . . A plant-based diet doesn't [necessarily] mean . . . a vegan diet."[8] EarthSave International advocates view the vegan diet as ideal; they simply see "plant-based" as a less-threatening term for the general public than "vegan." In addition to books, videotapes, and audiotapes produced by Robbins, EarthSave International publishes and distributes such brochures and booklets as "Our Food, Our World: The

Realities of an Animal-Based Diet" and "What's the Beef and Who Pays?" EarthSave also assists in the development of local groups, and in 1995, its Healthy School Lunch Program received an anonymous grant of almost three hundred thousand dollars to help introduce vegetarian foods into ten U.S. public school districts.[9]

VRG, which grew out of the local group Baltimore Vegetarians, founded by Charles Stahler and Debra Wasserman in 1982, is another organization that combines public outreach with efforts to change perceptions of vegetarianism in social institutions. By 1989, the group had so many members throughout North America that Stahler and Wasserman decided to change it from a local into a national organization. In addition to publishing several books, VRG publishes the bimonthly magazine *Vegetarian Journal* and three newsletters: *Tips for Activists* (for local groups and individual vegetarian activists), *VRG Update* (for significant donors), and *Food Service Update* (for food service personnel in public institutions, such as hospitals, schools, and government offices). The organization also holds a vegetarian essay contest for youths and sponsors booths at professional meetings held for dietitians and other health care workers. Although VRG acts as a resource to local groups and aspiring individual vegetarians, its primary focus is institutional change.

In 1986, Gene and Lorri Bauston founded the organization Farm Sanctuary, whose purpose (as set forth in the spring 1996 issue of its *Sanctuary News*) is to end "the exploitation of animals used for food production."[10] Farm Sanctuary rescues abused farm animals, documents incidents of farm animal abuse, encourages fast-food chains to add vegetarian options to their menus, and educates the public about vegetarian diets. In addition, the group worked to pass the 1995 Downed Animals Protection Act in California, which levies a fine against any farm owner convicted of leaving a disabled animal to die. The organization is now working to pass federal legislation (H.R. 453 and S. 850) that would require stockyards to euthanize critically ill and injured animals in a humane manner.[11]

More than seven hundred rescued animals live at the two Farm Sanctuary sites in Watkins Glen, New York, and Orland, California. These sanctuaries, which operate as education centers, provide daily tours and supply the public with such vegetarian information sheets as "The Beef with Beef," "Break the Egg Habit," and "The Problem with Pork." Farm Sanctuary is strongly affiliated with both the vegetarian and animal rights movements. Farm Sanctuary, FARM—both of which focus on the plight of farm animals and work to educate the public about the benefits of vegetarian diets—and Vegan Outreach are particularly concerned with promoting the ethical aspects of vegetarianism.

Grassroots Activist/Educational Organizations

FARM, Vegan Outreach, and Vegan Action are organizations that educate the general public and operate as educational centers for grassroots activists.

In 1981, Alex Hershaft—who had founded the Vegetarian Information Service in 1976 and had been active in NAVS—founded the group Farm Animal Reform Movement (FARM) as a task force at an animal rights conference in Allentown, Pennsylvania. Initially, FARM set out to achieve two goals: to reform the farm animal industry and to change consumer preferences. Today, however, the organization concentrates primarily on the latter goal, and as a result of this new focus, has dropped its full name in favor of the acronym. FARM organizes such campaigns as Veal Ban Action Day and the Great American Meat-Out, which encourage activists to work at the local level.

Vegan Action's "Join Us" brochure describes the group as "a grassroots activist network focused on promoting the vegan diet and lifestyle and inspiring more people to become actively involved in the vegan movement." The organization grew from a group of students at the University of California at Berkeley who organized to petition their school's Housing and Dining Services to offer a vegan entrée at every meal. After this successful effort, members began to design materials to help students at other colleges and universities conduct their own vegan dorm food campaigns.[12] Like many of the public outreach/educational organizations, Vegan Action plans to start organizing local chapters.

Vegan Outreach, founded in 1993, has a more missionary focus. The group publishes "Why Vegan?" a booklet describing the ethical basis of veganism. As cofounder Matt Ball explains the group's purpose, "We exist to reach people who might never learn what really goes on behind the scenes, and we provide resources and support to others around the country who are trying to do the same."[13] By March 1999, Vegan Outreach activists had distributed over six hundred thousand copies of the brochure, primarily by leafleting on college campuses. Vegan Outreach's website (see Appendix B), which includes such publications as "Tips for Promoting Veganism" and "Anger, Humor, and Advocacy," also helps educate future grassroots activists.

Several other smaller and less-visible groups operate at the national level, notably the Friends' Vegetarian Society, the Vegetarian Awareness Network (VEGANET), the Vegetarian Education Network, the North American Jewish Vegetarian Society, and Vegetarian Life (the vegetarian section of Mensa). These groups provide information through newsletters and other publications and sometimes concentrate on specific advocacy projects.

Characteristics of Local Vegetarian Groups

National vegetarian organizations spread their information locally through vegetarian groups in cities and towns throughout the United States and Canada. Many local vegetarian groups use national organization resources, inviting national representatives to speak and distributing their literature. To find out more about these groups, I conducted a survey between September 1995 and April 1996. The survey netted responses from ninety-seven active local vegetarian groups in the United States and Canada, eighty in the United States and seventeen in Canada.[14]

Because a major focus of many national organizations is to help create and nurture local groups, many local groups originate with contact between an individual and one of the national organizations. Sixty-one of the local groups surveyed claim affiliation with at least one national organization, most with NAVS, but this affiliation is often very loose. Affiliation with a national organization often allows members of the local group to receive discounted membership in the national organization and allows the local group to purchase discounted vegetarian books to resell at a profit. Only EarthSave International requires its affiliates to adopt a common statement of purpose.

Typically, when one or two people decide to start a local group, they organize a potluck dinner, a video showing, or a speaking engagement, which they then advertise in local health food stores and newspapers. The founders usually become the group's de facto leaders. Structured organization comes later, as the organization attracts more members. Of the groups surveyed, less than one-half (45 percent) have elected leaders, less than one-third (30 percent) have an elected board of directors, and 29 percent claim to have tax-exempt status. A majority (62 percent) publish monthly or quarterly newsletters to publicize their activities.

The primary function of local groups is to provide a sense of community among vegetarians in a particular region. Whereas some local vegetarian groups (29 percent) claim to have an entirely social function, other groups (71 percent) offer both public outreach and social support. The solely social groups typically have monthly potluck dinners or restaurant outings and occasional local speakers. They offer support to attendees and a way for them to share vegetarian foods and recipes. The many local vegetarian groups that offer some combination of social support for members and educational outreach to the general public set up tables to hand out literature at local festivals; offer cooking classes; organize library exhibits; or sponsor public festivals and dinners for World Vegetarian Day, the Great American Meat-Out, or Earth Day.

Only one group out of the ninety-seven surveyed, the VivaVegie Society in New York City, engages *solely* in public outreach and activist activities in its local area. Members of the VivaVegie Society regularly pass out literature on New York City streets, especially at festivals and parades. The group's purpose (according to the group's website—see Appendix B) is to "confront Mr. and Ms. Pedestrian to get the facts out about [a] healthful, ethical and environmentally conscious diet." The cornerstone of the VivaVegie Society, a four-page manifesto called "101 Reasons Why I'm a Vegetarian," lists facts about the benefits of a vegetarian diet; more than seventy thousand copies have been distributed. In 1999, the VivaVegie Society opened the Vegetarian Center of New York City, with a vegetarian news archive and information service.

Because the motivations for food choices can be many and varied, members of vegetarian groups often have little more than food in common. This may explain not only why the predominant activity of local vegetarian groups is sharing potluck meals but also why many local groups have difficulty finding volunteers and other resources. In the course of my survey, I received a great deal of correspondence from former organizers who seemed exasperated by members' lack of commitment. As one former leader of a local group in New York put it, "Our group has been reduced to a few couples who don't really want to do much, except eat and be merry." And as a former leader of a local group in California wrote, "After 3 years with no organizational help from other members, the leaders chose to stop and allow the group to either take over or let it drop. No one assumed the job and the group is no longer meeting." These responses concur with those in Akers's survey, which found that local vegetarian group organizers cited lack of leadership as their biggest problem.[15]

Although local groups may suffer from lack of both money and human resources, they reach the general public in ways that the national groups cannot. National groups act as clearinghouses of information, providing literature and support to local groups; local groups disseminate this information throughout their respective communities and offer the opportunity for person-to-person sharing of vegetarian foods and ideas.

Related and Overlapping Social Movements

The vegetarian movement does not exist in a vacuum. Other social movements and "civilizing" cultural trends contribute to an increasing interest in vegetarian diets.[16] In the 1960s, for example, the hippie movement generated concern about the use of animals for food.[17] On a larger and more amorphous scale, long-term cultural trends concerning bodily control and civility have led to an increased sensitivity about eating meat.[18] And other social causes, such as the animal rights, environmental, and health food movements, have helped change perceptions about how animals should be treated and whether they should be consumed as food.

The Animal Rights Movement

The North American animal rights movement focuses on the establishment of fundamental rights to life, liberty, and the pursuit of happiness for all nonhuman animals. The movement can be traced through a long history of animal protection causes, dating back to the founding of the American Society for the Prevention of Cruelty to Animals (ASPCA) in 1866.[19] Animal rightists, who advocate the abolition of the human use of animals, often disagree with animal welfarists, who promote policies that improve the conditions of the animals that humans currently use for research and for food. Between these two groups ideologically and strategically are the "pragmatists,"[20] who seek gradual replacement of the animals that humans use with nonanimal alternatives.

The vegetarian movement and the animal rights movement share some ideas, group structures, and members, but they operate primarily as two distinct movements. Although some large animal rights organizations, such as PETA and PCRM, make substantial efforts to promote veganism, most animal rights groups focus on promoting the rights of animals in experimental labs, zoos, and circuses (and only secondarily on farms).[21] At the same time, the mission statements of many vegetarian organizations include animal rights with concerns about personal and environmental health. Vegetarian groups use animal rights as one among many means of promoting vegetarianism.

Neither vegetarian and animal rights organizations nor their constituents are coterminous. Many animal rights activists (37 percent, according to one survey) are not vegetarians, and many vegetarians (85 percent, according to another survey) are not primarily motivated by a concern for animal rights.[22] Members of vegetarian organizations are less likely than members of animal rights organizations to approve of dramatic forms of activism (such as breaking into medical laboratories).[23] Because most vegetarians' initial motivation is their own personal health and they tend to become more committed to animal rights issues only gradually over time, organizational leaders and longtime vegetarians often share views in common with animal rights activists that newcomers do not. In addition, the vegetarian and animal rights movements typically mobilize new constituents differently:

Whereas animal rights organizations recruit strangers by administering "moral shocks" in the form of violently compelling literature and photographs, the vegetarian movement relies on "gentle" education, personal examples, and recruitment within social networks.[24] Although both movements address the fate of nonhuman animals, they do so by means of significantly different ideologies, organizational structures, and strategies.

The Health Food Movement

"Health foods" and "natural foods" generally refer to products grown without pesticides or chemicals. The concept of health foods dates back to the late nineteenth century, when Kellogg initiated the mass production of breakfast cereals, such as corn flakes and all-bran. Years later, the natural foods rage of the 1960s and 1970s led to a proliferation of health food stores and natural food co-ops.[25]

In the 1980s, large food corporations began to notice consumer interest in natural foods, and the mainstream food industry began to co-opt health food products. Food industry executives, for example, transformed granola from a breakfast meal into a snack food[26] (although in many cases, such new, "natural" products contain as much fat and calories as a chocolate candy bar). Meanwhile, the food industry also intensified its production of reduced-calorie, reduced-caffeine, higher-fiber foods. Sales of these products jumped more than 33 percent between 1985 and 1990.[27]

Profoundly diffuse, the health food movement is spread among organizations and industries and is held together primarily by small groups of people who practice a particular food philosophy or participate in food co-op activity. The Center for Science in the Public Interest, the Pure Food Campaign, and a few other interest groups seem to defend the merits of some health foods, but their goal is more to critique the unhealthful aspects of mainstream food production and consumption. The Kushi Institute (founded by Michio Kushi) and the Life Science Institute (founded by Harvey and Marilyn Diamond) are health food organizations that focus on education by providing literature and cooking classes to prospective adherents. And the National Health Association, formerly the American Natural Hygiene Society (a vegetarian natural food organization), promotes "the physiological and lifestyle practices that ensure health, happiness, peace and prosperity for everyone, everywhere."[28]

This limited formal organization within the health food movement is supplemented by communication distribution centers or "network nodes."[29] These sites include "health food stores, and restaurants, organic farms, . . . vegetarian food lines at schools,"[30] and food co-ops. Those who shop at health food stores are most likely to be well-educated females in their thirties or forties who are concerned about pursuing good nutrition and avoiding additives and preservatives. The vast majority of people who eat health and natural foods do not belong to any formal health food organization, although they may share a common worldview that celebrates purity, harmony, and nature.[31]

Organizations that promote healthful foods and healthful eating do not necessarily espouse vegetarianism. For example, although the Center for Science in the Public Interest accepts vegetarian diets as healthful, it gives positive evaluations of some meat products and publishes recipes that include meat. And health food industry spokespeople refer to organically grown beef as a health food. In addition, although health food regimens such as the Adele Davis Diet and macrobiotic diets are primarily vegetarian, they include occasional consumption of fish or other animal products. Similarly, even though a large percentage of vegetarians are motivated by health reasons, not all vegetarians eat health foods.[32] "Junk food vegetarians"—usually motivated by animal rights—may dine on soda, french fries, and Burger King's Veggie Whopper (a Whopper with everything but the beef).

The Environmental Movement

The vegetarian movement overlaps less with the environmental movement than with the animal rights and health food movements. In fact, the environmental movement might best be defined as *potentially* overlapping the vegetarian movement. Although environmentalists (especially radical environmentalists) may be more likely than the general population to follow vegetarian diets, environmental organizations are typically no more than minimally involved in promoting vegetarianism. In contrast, vegetarian leaders and groups promote environmental reasons for vegetarianism, even though only a small percentage of vegetarians are motivated primarily by environmental issues.[33] As we have noted, however, most vegetarian groups—with the notable exception of EarthSave International—address personal health benefits before presenting environmental reasons for vegetarianism.

The animal rights, health food, and environmental movements all share some common ground with the vegetarian movement. All attract some of the same adherents and share some beliefs about the deleterious effects of eating meat.

The Antivegetarian Countermovement

Current social movements include not only a vegetarian movement but also an antivegetarian countermovement. Although there are no explicitly antivegetarian organizations, meat industry organizations and other groups regularly critique vegetarian views. Vegetarianism has affected the meat industry and its supporters by moving their "taken-for-granted assumptions into the open, necessitating their justification and defense."[34] For the most part, instead of confronting vegetarianism directly, the meat industry has adapted its products to consumers' tastes, primarily by reducing fat contents and by promoting the health and flavor qualities of various meats. Beef and pork producers have tried to manage the public images of their products by launching campaigns such as "pork—the other white meat" and "beef—it's what's for dinner." According to the National Pork Producers Council's *Porkfolio of Lean Routines*, "In today's meat case, you'll find pork products with an average of 31% less fat, 29% less saturated fat, 10% less cholesterol and 14% fewer calories compared to 20 years ago."[35] Similarly, the beef industry has worked to provide the public with "extra lean" and "select" beef to meet the demand for lower-fat foods.[36]

As meat producers focus on making meats more palatable to a consumer base that clamors for low-fat foods,[37] reactions against vegetarian diets seem to be increasing. Industry organizations such as the National Cattlemen's Beef Association (NCBA) and the Meat and Livestock Board have published reports that address vegetarian issues. A paper entitled "Myths and Facts about Vegetarianism" and a point-by-point critique of Robbins's *Diet for a New America*, for example, can be found on the NCBA website.[38] Similarly, the American Council on Science and Health (ACSH) published a critique of Jeremy Rifkin's *Beyond Beef* (which outlines the large-scale environmental and health consequences of the beef industry); its website also includes a scathing critique of vegetarianism.[39]

The meat industry also reacts, and has been known to get results, when vegetarianism receives positive media attention. For example, when the NCBA protested a cover of *Muse* (the Smithsonian Institution's children's magazine) that featured a picture of a calf pleading, "Please don't eat me," the management reassigned the issue's editor and promised to feature letters from ranchers' children in a subsequent issue.[40] The meat industry also stepped up its beef promotion and publicly criticized vegetarianism when the mayor of Calgary, Alberta,

Canada, signed his local vegetarian society's meat-out proclamation. And, in perhaps the most notable of all vegetarian-related cases, a group of Texas cattle ranchers sued Oprah Winfrey, her production company (Harpo Productions), and vegetarian activist Howard Lyman for making allegedly disparaging remarks about beef on "The Oprah Winfrey Show."

"Tempest in a Feed-Lot": A Controversial World Vegetarian Month Proclamation in Calgary

On October 1, 1995, Al Duerr—mayor of Calgary, Alberta, Canada—signed (and issued a press release with) the following proclamation:

> During October, the Calgary Vegetarian Society will sponsor special events focusing on the benefits of a vegetarian lifestyle. This is an ideal opportunity for interested Calgarians to learn about vegetarianism.
>
> Whereas: Communities around the world will be celebrating World Vegetarian Day on October 1;
>
> Whereas: Several scientific studies have determined that a vegetarian diet can benefit one's health and help prevent disease;
>
> Whereas: Vegetarianism continues to gain interest around the world.
>
> On behalf of City Council and the citizens of Calgary, I hereby declare the month of October 1995 as:
>
> "Vegetarian Month"

Coincidentally, the Canada Beef Export Federation was meeting in Alberta when the mayor's office issued this proclamation.[41] After a reporter solicited opinions on the statement, members began to call the federation to object, and one Saskatchewan business sponsored twenty radio announcements promoting red meat. This is perhaps not surprising in light of the fact that the province of Alberta produces about 60 percent of Canada's beef,[42] and Calgary, which is also known as Cowtown, boasts a white cowboy hat as its symbol.

According to Alberta Cattle Commission Chairman Ben Thorlakson, "It is inconsistent for Calgary to support a vegetarian way of life."[43]

Four days after signing the proclamation, Mayor Duerr, who was up for reelection on October 16, issued a press release that stated, "The proclamation has been interpreted as promoting the exclusion of all meat, poultry and fish from the diet and has subsequently created significant controversy in the community. Therefore, Mayor Duerr has decided to rescind the proclamation."

Calgary Vegetarian Society (CVS) member Don Monroe coined the controversy a "tempest in a feed-lot"; in fact, according to CVS spokesperson Val Fitch, many people heard about the group for the first time during the controversy.[44] Not two months after Mayor Duerr (who had since been reelected) rescinded the proclamation, CVS had increased its paying membership by 40 percent, showing 260 members. In 1996, the mayor's office refused to make a World Vegetarian Day proclamation; a spokesperson stated, "When a subject is controversial, the conditions which make a proclamation acceptable no longer exist."[45] The Calgary "tempest in a feed-lot" made vegetarianism "controversial" and newsworthy, ultimately bringing more resources to the CVS and perhaps introducing more individuals to the concept of vegetarianism.

Mad Cow Disease, Oprah, and Food Disparagement

An even more dramatic reaction from the beef industry came in response to the April 16, 1996, "Oprah Winfrey Show" program on bovine spongiform encephalopathy (BSE), or mad cow disease.[46] On the program, Howard Lyman, former cattle rancher and current president of EarthSave International, debated representatives from the NCBA and the USDA about the safety of the U.S. beef supply. After Lyman described the process by which some diseased cows are processed into feed for other cows, Winfrey proclaimed, "It has just stopped me *cold* from eating another burger!" The program aired in Chicago five minutes before live cattle futures were to be traded at the Chicago Mercantile Exchange, and, with the prediction that consumers would cut back on beef purchases as a result of the show, prices dropped dramatically.

Several states (thirteen in 2001), including Texas, have food product disparagement laws that make it illegal to knowingly lodge false or misleading claims about the healthfulness or safety of a food product.[47] On the basis of these laws, beef industry and agricultural representatives encouraged attorney generals in several states to lodge product disparagement lawsuits against Lyman (who stated that "BSE will make AIDS look like the common cold"), Oprah Winfrey, and Winfrey's Harpo Productions; a group of Texas cattle ranchers then sued them and went to trial in Amarillo, Texas, in early 1998.[48] Because only perishable food products are protected under the Texas statute and the judge deemed that cattle are not perishable food products, the defendants were ultimately acquitted.[49]

Although Oprah, Lyman, and Harpo Productions were all cleared of the charges, the trial has not led to an increase in free speech about meat production; in fact, some claim that the reverse is true. Fear of prolonged litigation and enormous court costs may well inhibit activists, educators, and other citizens from speaking out about food problems and industry interests. These fears may not be unfounded. In 1999, inspired in part by a PETA billboard in Amarillo that stated, "Jesus was a vegetarian," the beef industry stepped up its efforts to track derogatory comments about its products. To educate critics, the Texas and Southwestern Cattle Raisers Association set up a hotline to receive reports of disparaging remarks. According to Rob Hosford, association spokesperson, the hotline focuses on comments by critics in the news media: "If we hear XYZ radio station carrying something about the beef industry, procedures and products that is derogatory, unfounded and untrue, with this task force we will send someone over there to re-educate, so the next time they talk they'll be talking from the right side of the ballpark."[50] As the beef industry steps up its surveillance, we can expect more lengthy and costly food disparagement trials in the future.

Clearly, then, when its interests are directly threatened, the beef industry publicly confronts vegetarian interests. Barring these circumstances, however, the meat industry tends to downplay the prevalence of vegetarianism and focus on promotion of the positive qualities of meat. If vegetarian issues increasingly find their way into public discussion, we can expect more frequent and more direct attacks of the movement by the meat industry. This may prove to be a blessing in disguise, however, since such controversies focus more attention on meat eating as a health and social issue and give the vegetarian movement a rare opportunity to have its viewpoints heard.

The Vegetarian Movement: Thriving, Wilting, or Maintaining?

The vegetarian movement's primary concerns are to motivate individuals to become vegetarians, increase the cultural acceptance of vegetarianism, and make vegetarian foods more readily available. Although relatively few vegetarians belong to formal organizations, these groups play an important role in (1) articulating the meanings associated with the vegetarian way of life and (2) spreading these meanings by providing materials to local groups and grassroots activists and by sponsoring conferences and other activities. All national vegetarian groups engage in public outreach, but some also focus on institutional change within the educational system and the health professions.

Each national organization has its own set of projects, and—aside from publicizing one another's activities and occasionally attending one another's conferences—groups share few activities and campaigns in common. This lack of mutual activities is perhaps partly attributable to some long-standing personality and ideological conflicts,[51] but lack of resources (both human and monetary) is also a major problem. For example, at the 1995 Vegetarian Summerfest (a national conference sponsored by NAVS), several national group leaders discussed the possibility of forming a Better Foods Council, an interest group that would counter the meat and dairy industries and promote vegetarian diets. Several leaders considered this to be a good project in theory, but time and other resource constraints thwarted early efforts to create the coalition. Lack of committed, active members and lack of money often prevent vegetarian organizations from engaging in publicly visible campaigns that promote vegetarianism. In general, national vegetarian organizations do not seem to be expanding their membership, and since 1990, only two relatively small grassroots activist–oriented national organizations, Vegan Outreach and Vegan Action (both geared toward college students), have formed. Perhaps this suggests the wave of the future: Most vegetarian organizations are maintaining their membership and activities levels, as growth occurs within groups that cater to teenagers and college students.

Animal rights organizations constitute a significant part of the vegetarian social movement field. Even though they devote much of their resources to activities that protect animal rights in other arenas, large animal rights organizations such as PCRM and PETA have embarked on more-massive vegetarian (primarily vegan) campaigns than have vegetarian organizations. These organizations, as noted at the beginning of this chapter, count members in the hundreds of thousands.

One explanation for the comparative success of the animal rights movement in attracting a paying membership is that its direct-mail campaigns—which highlight the most extreme atrocities that involve animal suffering—evoke a more intense response in vulnerable recipients than do vegetarian campaigns. Although some vegetarian organizations offer as a feature of membership publications that are not widely available elsewhere,[52] most national vegetarian groups, when compared with national animal rights organizations, offer potential members educational material that is less likely to inspire them, and their message generally carries less ethical urgency.

4 Vegetarianism

*Expressions of Ideology
in Vegetarian Organizations*

It makes a difference whether vegetarianism is a "diet" or a "phil-osophy." A diet is a list of the foods you choose—a philosophy is a set of coherent REASONS for making those choices. You cannot build a movement around a "diet." To have a movement you have to have people believing, living and working in concert to realize an ideal.
—Stanley Sapon, "What's in a Name?"

Vegetarianism, the movement's ideology, criticizes meat eating and offers a vision for a meatless world; it is a set of ideas and values that people and organizations can draw from and combine in different ways. In his early treatment of social movements, sociologist Herbert Blumer defined ideology as "a body of doctrine, beliefs, and myths" that gives a move-ment "direction, justification, weapons of attack, weapons of defense, and inspiration and hope."[1] As such, an ideology is a symbolic system that people construct and manipulate, a set of interrelated meanings that may make sense to one group of people but not another. An ideology serves multiple purposes for any social movement. For example, it provides both mean-ing and direction to social movement participants, giving them a sense of purpose and the momentum to act. Outside of the movement, an ideology can attract and mobilize new members, functioning as an organization's "calling card" to reach the general public.[2] Expressions of ideology, then, can

70

both increase commitment within a movement and attract new members.

Like all social movement ideologies, vegetarianism is a multifaceted, multilayered set of ideas. The concept includes three basic tenets: compassion for all living beings, the health and vitality of vegetarian diets, and concern for the environment.[3] Advocates and movement leaders sometimes debate the finer points of vegetarianism (for example, does honey harvesting cause bees to suffer?), but—because the ideology reflects a long-standing interconnected system of beliefs and ideas to which longtime vegetarians and newcomers alike refer for justification of their practices—they rarely contest its basic tenets. Instead, vegetarian leaders are more likely to debate *how* these tenets of the ideology should be presented to potential adherents.

The general approach for presenting vegetarianism to the public can best be described as ecumenical. That is, although leaders and their respective organizations may stress one or more tenets over others, most embrace all of the tenets of vegetarianism. Because they want to reach the broadest possible audience, they avoid the risk of alienating any particular group by promoting health, animal rights, or environmental issues exclusively.

The Basic Tenets of Vegetarianism

Vegetarianism is rooted in basic ideas about the ideal relationships between humans and their social and physical environments; it expresses an ideal state of nature in which health and happiness are linked with caring and compassion for others.

Compassion for All Living Beings

The concern for living creatures is embodied in the ancient concepts of ahimsa (nonviolence), from Eastern religions

(Jainism, Buddhism, and Hinduism), and reverence for life, a concept promoted by Albert Schweitzer in the early 1900s.[4] Similarly, in the sixth century B.C., Pythagoras emphasized a vegetable diet in order to rekindle the connection with the natural world; he viewed all creatures as interconnected and equal, emphasizing that nonhuman animals were as capable as humans of possessing souls and virtues.[5] All of these philosophies support the idea that by consuming animals, we introduce into our bodies the fear and suffering that the animals experienced in death.

In 1970s popular discourse, people began to articulate concerns about nonviolence toward animals in terms of rights. The term "animal rights," which can be traced to philosopher Tom Regan's writings,[6] refers to equal moral status for all creatures that "are conscious [and] possess a complex awareness and a psychophysical identity over time";[7] human and nonhuman creatures have an inherent value that cannot be measured hierarchically. Consequently, a nonhuman animal is undeserving of any ill treatment that would be considered inappropriate for a human (such as hunting him or her or eating his or her flesh). Although the term "animal rights" has a very specific meaning, in popular discourse it has been watered down to refer to a general concern for animal welfare and well-being.

Where Regan's writings inspired debates among philosophers and activists, Peter Singer's *Animal Liberation: A New Ethic for Our Treatment of Animals,* sparked increasingly widespread dialogue about the moral status of animals; by 1988, more than 250,000 copies were in print.[8] *Animal Liberation* takes the position that the interests of animals deserve consideration equal to the interests of humans. According to Singer, equality among creatures should be based not on *identity* (the creature's apparent similarity to humans) but on the creature's capacity for suffering. He rejects René Descartes's view of animals as machines and softens the boundary between humans and animals by using the terms "human animals" and "nonhuman animals."

Singer draws parallels between racism, sexism, and speciesism (he defines "speciesism" as "a prejudice of attitude or bias toward the interests of members of one's own species and against those members of other species"): "To protest about bull-fighting in Spain or the slaughter of baby seals in Canada while continuing to eat chickens that have spent their lives crammed in cages, or veal from calves that have been deprived of their mothers, their proper diet, and the freedom to lie down with their legs extended, is like denouncing apartheid in South Africa while asking your neighbors not to sell their homes to blacks."[9] In Singer's view, anyone who opposes animal cruelty should become a vegan. And anyone who claims to be an animal lover yet consumes meat is as much of a hypocrite as someone who publicly denounces racism but privately discriminates.

Similarly, Carol Adams and Marjorie Spiegel draw analogies between speciesism and other forms of prejudice.[10] In *The Sexual Politics of Meat*, Adams links animals' rights and women's rights; she argues that meat is "a symbol and celebration of male dominance" and that "to remove meat is to threaten the structure of the larger patriarchal culture."[11] Men objectify, fragment, and consume both women and animals in the parallel activities of sexual violence and butchering.[12] For Adams, this is not just an analogy; it is a causal relationship: By consuming meat, people reinforce both speciesism and patriarchal values.

In *The Dreaded Comparison: Human and Animal Slavery*, Spiegel juxtaposes the life and death experiences of factory-farmed animals and slaves. Like Singer and Adams, she asserts that when oppression of any kind is permitted, powerful groups and individuals can make arbitrary decisions about who should be dominated: "Any oppression helps to prop up other forms of oppression. This is why it is vital to link oppressions in our minds, to look for the common shared aspects and fight against them as one, rather than prioritizing victims' suffering."[13] Like Regan, Spiegel suggests that the inherent moral value of creatures should not be ranked.

Health and Vitality Associated with Vegetarian Diets

Another basic tenet of vegetarianism focuses on the life-giving quality of plant-based foods and the life-taking quality of meat products.[14] The word "vegetarian" is not a condensed version of "vegetable eater"; rather, it derives from the Latin *vegetus*, meaning "whole, sound, fresh, and lively."[15] Claims about the healthfulness of vegetarian diets date back to Pythagorean philosophy in the sixth century B.C.[16] Dating back to the Jacksonian health reformers and the early Seventh Day Adventists of the 1800s, this tenet has predominated the course of the North American vegetarian movement.

Vegetarians characterize plant foods as vital and meat products as dead or decaying. For example, in *What's Wrong with Eating Meat?* Barbara Parham writes, "Many plants retain their life-giving energy for many days after they remain still capable of sprouting and growing. Meat, on the other hand, has been in the process of decay for several days."[17] Moreover, meat takes longer than most vegetarian foods to pass through the intestinal tract, leaving the consumer feeling heavy.[18] Following a vegetarian diet can help alleviate this feeling, according to "Vegetarianism . . . a Diet for Life," a 1993 NAVS brochure written by Stanley Sapon, F. Berg, and L. Campanile: "You may be less constipated. People who eat a typical American diet may be constipated and not realize it. . . . Most new vegetarians report that they feel great! Some say they've never felt better in their lives. For some people, there is a very brief adjustment period where they may feel weak or tired. . . . Many do not experience this adjustment at all and most find after they adjust that they have more energy and feel better than ever." The health tenet of vegetarianism focuses on the positive, enlivening qualities of vegetarian foods. In fact, vegetarian authors note that vegetarians are less likely than meat eaters to suffer from a variety of diseases and ailments, including cancer, atherosclerosis, kidney disease, gout, arthritis, digestion and elimination problems, asthma, anemia, gallstones, hypoglycemia, and diabetes.

In vegetarianism, the health and ethical tenets interact in that a vegetarian diet is thought to make a person more peaceful and less violent. In other words, not only does vegetarianism *exemplify* nonviolence; it also *causes* it. The claim that meat eating leads to the embodiment of violence extends the aphorism "You are what you eat": One who eats violence becomes violent. This concept also dates back to Pythagoras, who linked vegetarianism with peacefulness and pacifism.[19] Recent authors such as Robbins express this idea as well: "When we eat animals who have died violent deaths we literally eat their fear. We take in biochemical agents designed by nature to tell an animal that its life is in the gravest danger, and it must either fight or flee for its life. And then in our wars and daily lives, we give expression to the panic in which the animals we have eaten died. . . . A nonviolent world has roots in a non-violent [*sic*] diet."[20] Similarly, Victoria Moran talks about the "phenomenon of 'pain poisoning'" that occurs when an animal is slaughtered under duress,[21] and she refers to an "indivisibility of violence" in which the violence of slaughter both indicates and inflames violence in other areas of life. And Rudolph Ballentine suggests that meat eating may "create inclinations to inexplicable violence or a pervasive sense of pointless anger and hostility."[22]

Advocates hold not only that eating a healthful, nonviolent diet creates a more moral person but also that practicing vegetarianism for ethical reasons provides health benefits. In *For the Vegetarian in You*, Billy Ray Boyd writes, "The inconvenience of reconditioning our taste buds is minor compared to the suffering we thereby relieve, and we are compensated with better health and a clearer conscience."[23] Similarly, in *Animal Factories,* Jim Mason and Peter Singer state, "The food you consume three or more times daily is your most constant and intimate connection with the environment and the living world around you. If you reflect your concerns for them in your food habits, you will be healthier in every way."[24] The potential positive consequences of vegetarianism and the potential negative consequences of meat eating are usually expressed in terms of individual health; however, a growing tendency to express these effects in terms of the societal costs of health care and decreased human output brings an additional moral component to the health argument for vegetarianism.[25]

Concern for the Environment

The third tenet of vegetarianism centers on the deleterious environmental effects of meat production and the food shortages that they create. Lappé first addressed this basis of vegetarianism in 1971 in *Diet for a Small Planet,* when she stated that "an acre of cereals can produce *five times* more protein than an acre devoted to meat production; legumes (peas, beans, lentils) can produce *ten times* more; leafy vegetables *fifteen times* more."[26] This tenet focuses on the waste of natural resources that results from meat production. Advocates contend that meat production depletes water supplies, forests, and fossil fuel energy and causes soil erosion. For example, writes Boyd, "a typical mixed plant and animal food diet requires about 2500 gallons of water *per day* to produce, compared with 300 gallons for a plant-based vegan diet."[27] Similarly, writes Akers, "over 90% of all agricultural land . . . is devoted to the production of animal products."[28] Advocates also argue that vegetable matter used to feed animals produced for meat could feed the hungry directly. According to Robbins, "If Americans reduced their meat consumption by

10 percent, enough grain would be saved to feed sixty million people."[29]

Ideological works tend to emphasize how the three distinct sets of arguments that ground vegetarianism reinforce one another. Robbins compares vegetarianism to a slot machine when all three pictures line up (animal rights, health, and concern for the environment): "The food choices that are healthiest for you . . . are best for the earth."[30] Although, as we have noted, vegetarian groups often initially promote the health benefits of a vegetarian diet, organization leaders generally encourage gradual adoption of *all* the ideological tenets of vegetarianism. In this way, adherents become more committed to the vegetarian ideal (often moving from ovo-lacto-vegetarianism to veganism) and thus more likely to advocate vegetarianism to others.

Vegetarianism and Veganism

Historically, "vegetarian" has been an umbrella term that includes not only those who follow lacto-, ovo-, and ovo-lacto-vegetarian diets but also those who follow the vegan diet and lifestyle. Today, however, vegetarianism is often equated with ovo-lacto-vegetarianism, and veganism is viewed as a completely separate category. Vegans are distinguished from "total vegetarians," who eat no animal foods or by-products yet use nonedible animal by-products such as leather and wool. Vegans avoid the use of all animal-derived foods (including dairy products, eggs, lactose, casein, whey, usually honey, and sometimes sugar)[31] and other products (including leather, wool, fur, and silk). Vegans view their lifestyle as the natural, logical consequence of the vegetarian arguments. Advocates who promote veganism primarily tend to focus on the concern for animals, particularly the suffering that dairy cows and laying hens experience. For example, in *A Vegetarian Sourcebook*, Akers—a longtime vegetarian advocate and president of the Colorado Vegetarian Society—writes, "Animals who provide dairy products and eggs suffer just as much—if not more—than animals raised specifically for slaughter, and most dairy cows and laying hens wind up at the slaughterhouse anyway. . . . Once one admits that what suffering animals experience while they are still alive is an important ethical issue, it is hard to escape the total vegetarian or vegan position."[32] Although veganism tends to center on the ethical dimensions of food consumption, the previous chapter illustrated some of the growing discussion about the negative *health* effects of dairy products.

As a result of a split among British vegetarians,[33] in 1944, Donald Watson coined the term "veganism" to distinguish it from other forms of vegetarianism. Some animosity between British vegetarians and vegans lingers to this day. In contrast, North American vegetarian leaders have witnessed minimal tension. According to Akers, "In Britain there's been sort of this antagonism, on ideological grounds. . . . whereas in the United States that's not present. Basically, there's a *quid pro quo* in the U.S and Canada. And that is that the vegetarians have allowed the vegans to take over their organizations. But, they have to *remain* vegetarian organizations and they have to allow lacto-ovo[-vegetarianism] as an alternative."[34] In the North American vegetarian movement, nearly all of the national organization leaders are vegans, but many promote a gradual path to vegetarianism that begins with ovo-lacto-vegetarianism. Although organization leaders sometimes disagree about how to *promote* vegetarianism and whether the word "vegan" should be used to attract new members, even leaders of the overtly vegan groups (Vegan Action, Vegan Outreach) resist criticizing the groups that avoid the "v word."

Vegetarianism in Organizations

Choosing to emphasize a particular aspect of vegetarianism is an organizational strategy that can generate consequences for the vegetarian ideology. When organizations create strategies based on one ideological dimension, the reinforcement of that particular tenet may cause it to become more prominent in the vegetarian system of beliefs. For example, EarthSave International promotes vegetarianism on ecological grounds; if, as a result of their efforts, an increasing number of people adopt vegetarianism for environmental reasons, this value may become more pronounced in vegetarian messages produced by other vegetarian organizations and advocates.

With the exception of EarthSave International, which promotes "plant-based" diets, vegetarian organizations promote all vegetarian diets or only the vegan diet and lifestyle. Although all the leaders of national-level organizations that I interviewed are vegans—who typically espouse veganism for reasons that reflect a combination of the basic tenets of vegetarianism—vegetarian organizations do not necessarily adopt strategies based on the leaders' personal preferences. They consider instead which aspects of vegetarianism are most likely to attract new adherents.

Public Outreach/Educational Organizations

In their presentations of ideology, organizations that focus on public outreach and education use an ecumenical approach that often focuses on health issues. The NAVS mission statement, for example, declares simply, "Founded in 1974, the North American Vegetarian Society is a non-profit educational organization dedicated to promoting the vegetarian way of life."[35] Every issue of the NAVS quarterly periodical *Vegetarian Voice* carries the subtitle "Perspectives on Healthy, Ecological, and Compassionate Living." The magazine contains many health-related articles and recipes and also addresses animal rights and environmental issues. For its annual public conference (Vegetarian Summerfest), NAVS invites speakers who approach vegetarianism from different ideological viewpoints.

Like NAVS, VUNA advocates an ecumenical approach to vegetarianism that embraces all of the ideology's tenets. By strengthening local vegetarian groups, VUNA seeks to accomplish its mission "to promote a strong, effective, cooperative vegetarian movement throughout North America."[36]

Although, more than NAVS and VUNA, AVS focuses on the ethical bases of vegetarianism, the group's periodical, *Ahimsa,* publishes many health-related flyers and articles. With its fall 1996 newsletter, AVS sent a handout entitled "Alternatives to Dairy Products and Eggs," along with fifty vegan recipes. The AVS mission statement as set forth in *Ahimsa* states, "The American Vegan Society is a non-profit, non-sectarian, non-political, tax-exempt educational membership organization teaching a compassionate way of living according to Ahimsa and Reverence for Life."

Leaders of public outreach/educational organizations seem to adopt an ecumenical approach that can draw a wide audience and minimize the conflicts that might arise among members who embrace vegetarianism for different reasons.

Institutional Change/Educational Organizations

Although organizations that focus on institutional change and education tend to emphasize a particular vegetarian tenet of choice, these groups also adopt an ecumenical approach. For example, the VRG mission statement—as set forth in the group's periodical *Vegetarian Journal*—states, "We are a non-profit organization which educates the public about vegetarianism and the interrelated issues of health, nutrition, ecology, ethics, and world hunger." Even so, however, VRG leaders described their organization to the 1996 Vegetarian Summerfest audience as a "vegan, activist-oriented group."[37] *Vegetarian Journal* and other VRG publications focus predominantly on health and nutrition issues. In accordance, the organization seeks institutional change in nutrition-related areas, such as altering federal School Lunch Program guidelines, and gaining acceptance from the ADA and other professional organizations.

Similarly, EarthSave International, which focuses largely on environmental issues, also espouses an ecumenical ideology. The organization's mission statement, as presented in its newsletter, states:

> EarthSave is dedicated to helping create a better world by showing the powerful impacts of our ordinary eating habits and promoting positive alternatives. We educate people about the dietary link to environmental degradation, encouraging sound nutrition, conservation of resources and sustainable agriculture. We show how an animal-based diet, and the factory farming which underlies it, causes enormous depletion and pollution of the natural world, suffering for the animals, and danger to our own health.

Farm Sanctuary actively promotes the animal rights tenet of the vegetarian ideology as it increasingly addresses the health benefits of veganism. According to the organization's mission statement, as given in its newsletter, "Farm Sanctuary is a national non-profit organization dedicated to ending the exploitation of animals used for food production." By inviting people to visit rescued animals at Farm Sanctuary shelters in New York and California, the group works to focus people's attention on the methods of meat production and their effect on farm animals.

In their efforts to effect institutional change, VRG, Earth-Save, and Farm Sanctuary adopt an ecumenical approach, even as they focus on a single ideological tenet (health, environment, or animal rights).

Grassroots Activist/Educational Organizations

Grassroots activist/educational groups focus mostly on animal concerns and take an approach that is less explicitly ecumenical than that of their public outreach counterparts. The leaders of both FARM and Vegan Outreach consider their organizations to be part of both the animal rights and vegetarian movements.

According to the mission statement set forth in FARM's newsletter, the group is "a national, non-profit, public-interest organization" formed in 1981 by animal, consumer, and environmental protection advocates to expose and stop animal abuse and other destructive impacts of factory farming. FARM focuses on the animal rights tenet of the vegetarian ideology and has recently switched its target audience from producers to consumers. With this shift, FARM expanded its original ideology from a nearly exclusive focus on animal rights to an ideology that includes the tenets of health and environment.[38]

Vegan Outreach's mission statement, as presented in the organization's newsletter, identifies the group's commitment to animal rights: "Vegan Outreach's philosophy is that each sentient animal has a right to his or her body and life. To that end, Vegan Outreach promotes the lifestyle of veganism—living so as to contribute to as little exploitation and death as possible." Vegan Outreach's booklet, "Why Vegan?" which it distributes widely on college campuses, also addresses health and environmental reasons for veganism.

Local Organizations

With the exception of EarthSave local groups, which must adopt the EarthSave statement of purpose (see Chapter 3), all nationally affiliated and nonaffiliated groups are free to adopt or do without mission statements of their own. Earth-Save groups excluded, only about one-half (53 percent) of the local vegetarian groups in my survey use a formal mission statement. Because a formal statement of purpose reflects a negotiated commitment among members to share common purposes and goals, this statistic suggests a lack of formal organization among these groups.

Like national groups, local vegetarian societies tend to present ecumenical ideologies that embrace all the tenets of vegetarianism. The following are some examples:

- The mission statement of the Corning Area Vegetarian Society in New York, as set forth in its newsletter, "Food for Thought," is as follows: "The Corning Area Vegetarian Society is a non-profit, non-sectarian association whose goal is to promote the health, ethical, and ecological benefits of vegetarianism. We welcome all vegetarians, as well as those who may not yet be vegetarian but are interested in learning more."
- The mission statement of the Gulf Coast Vegetarian Society in Florida, as presented in its brochure by the same name, is as follows: "The Gulf Coast Vegetarian Society is a group of individuals who believe that a vegetarian diet is essential in attaining personal health, global health and the well-being of animals. We share a concern for one or all of these issues and offer support to anyone who wishes to follow a vegetarian diet."
- The mission statement of the Vegetarians of Oklahoma City, as stated on a response to my survey, is as follows: "Vegetarians of Oklahoma City are committed to promoting vegetarianism in our community through education, interaction, and mutual support. We believe that the reduced consumption of animal products promotes healthier lives, environmental conservation and compassion to all life on the planet. We welcome vegetarians and non-vegetarians alike."

In addition to reflecting all the tenets of vegetarianism, these expressions of ideology reflect an inclusive approach to membership that embraces vegetarians and nonvegetarians alike.

Boundary Work and Vegetarianism

Advocates often articulate ideology in public—what can also be called the "front stage" of social movement activity—using its tenets as promotional tools to attract new members. Therefore, when vegetarian leaders consider changing how vegetarianism is presented, they take into account the reactions they might receive from the public.

The give-and-take of these discussions—which is carried out at vegetarian conferences and through e-mail discussion groups—is important because of the strong interconnection between a social movement's ideology and its strategies; choosing a particular tenet affects the strategies that leaders enact. Any of the ideological tenets may open the possibility of using some strategies and close or limit the possibility of using others. If an organization emphasizes the health component of vegetarianism, for example, it is unlikely that the group will promote vegetarianism by wearing "I don't eat my friends" T-shirts. At the same time, organizational leaders are aware that articulating a particular ideological tenet may attract some audiences and repel others. Some people may consider PETA's "Jesus was a vegetarian" campaign a thought-provoking way of pointing to the ethics of meat eating, for example, whereas others may find it somewhat objectionable or even sacrilegious.

Historically, a vegetarian has been defined simply in terms of diet—someone who avoids meat, poultry, and seafood with or without the inclusion of eggs and dairy products—without regard for the particular reason(s) that he or she chooses this practice. A person may become a vegetarian for any reason or combination of reasons discussed herein or for no ideological reason at all. Consequently, as one local group leader said to me, "The only thing we have is common is what we *don't* do."[39]

Also historically, a vegan diet has been regarded as one vegetarian option, coexisting with lacto-, ovo-, and ovo-lacto-vegetarian diets. "Vegetarian" has been the umbrella term that describes all of these. Although organizations have traditionally presented vegetarian ideology in a straightforward ecumenical way that often emphasizes the health component, recently there has been a movement to change the definition of vegetarianism to reflect an explicitly ethical focus and to clarify that veganism, rather than being a subset of vegetarianism, is the natural and desired lifestyle for all vegetarians. Although it is not yet clear whether this debate signifies the advent of a major shift in leaders' public definition of vegetarianism or a minor rift among ideologues, the controversy demonstrates leaders' concern about the role and strategic consequences of ideology in vegetarian organizations.

The movement to change the definition of vegetarianism began at the 1996 Vegetarian Summerfest. There Stanley Sapon (an emeritus professor of linguistics at the University of Rochester) presented a paper entitled "What's in a Name? Vegetarianism's Past, Present, and Future: A Linguistic and Behavioral Appraisal."[40] According to the NAVS, this presentation "drew a standing ovation and launched the beginning of an international dialogue about the real meaning of vegetarianism."[41] Sapon proposed, and encouraged all vegetarian groups to consider and accept, the following definition: "Vegetarianism is a philosophy that manifests its reverence and respect for the well-being of all sentient life by advocating and striving for the ultimate adoption of a plant-based diet."[42]

According to Sapon, the current definition of vegetarianism suggests a hierarchy in which an ovo-lacto-vegetarian diet can be construed as less "advanced" than a vegan diet: "In this verbal climate [of a hierarchy of preferable diets] it is impossible to avoid the implication that vegan is higher on the scale . . . better, and ovo-lacto is lower and not as good. At this point the notion of 'holier than Thou' makes its appearance, and an inevitable foundation of discordant—sometimes corrosive—divisiveness is laid down."[43] Still, for Sapon, veganism should be the ultimate ideal, not just one of many vegetarian options. And he views conventional vegetarian wisdom that prescribes a sequence for the elimination of animal products (meat first, then eggs and dairy products) as inconsistent, because it suggests that eggs and dairy products are more morally acceptable than meat: "Regardless of one's personal dietary custom, given what we know about the way milk is produced, it is a frank breach of ethics to suggest to the uninformed that while the flesh of a cow is unacceptable as human food, the milk of that cow is [acceptable]."[44] In other words, Sapon wants to eliminate both the perceived hierarchical division between ovo-lacto-vegetarians and vegans and the perception that dairy products and eggs are morally acceptable meat alternatives.

Presumably, Sapon's use of the term "plant-based diet" is intended to further soften the potentially conflictual division between ovo-lacto-vegetarians and vegans. As we have noted, EarthSave International uses this term, as do FARM, NAVS, Vegan Action, and other groups. In addition, some vegetarian authors use the term "plant-based diet," particularly when they fear that the "v" words ("vegetarian" and "vegan") may seem too radical in a particular context.

Within several months of the presentation, says Sapon, "there [was] a flood of reaction that I . . . heard in person, [by] phone, and [by] mail, and a continuing stream of comment and dialogue in over a hundred postings on the internet,"[45] suggesting that, indeed, his words had sparked dialogue in the movement, with leaders and adherents both defending and attacking the new definition. Numerous Internet postings about Sapon's presentation appeared on vegetarian discussion lists, most of which did not favor Sapon's redefinition. Although Sapon indicates that he wishes vegetarianism to be inclusive of all types of vegetarians, many viewed his definition as exclusive rather than inclusive, and potentially alienating to newcomers. Specifically, they perceived exclusion of people who follow vegetarian diets (whether ovo-lacto-vegetarian or vegan) solely for health reasons (or for any reasons other than ethics) and inclusion of semivegetarians who aspire to the goal of adopting a totally plant-based diet. In other words, they interpreted Sapon's definition as based on *intention* and *motivation* to follow a vegan diet, rather than on actual dietary practice.

According to Akers, this muddles the already confusing definition of what constitutes a vegetarian: "It ignores the more serious threat against the meaning of the term 'vegetarian': the overwhelming number of people who are self-described vegetarians actually eat meat. . . . Shouldn't this be sending shock waves through the vegetarian community? Shouldn't we be redoubling our efforts to make clear that vegetarians don't eat chicken and fish?"[46]

Some vegetarian advocates have also expressed concern that Sapon's definition gives the impression that prospective vegetarians must ultimately live up to the vegan ideal, thus scaring away potential members. Sapon disagrees. In an epilogue to his presentation, he once again stresses the importance of minimizing the conflict between the different types of vegetarians and the need for a common purpose: "When vegetarian groups are led by a vegan 'elite' who feel obliged to protect their ovo-lacto members from any suggestions that their food choices are less than ideal, it is more than patronizing—it saps the vitality from the movement and paralyzes it."[47] Sapon argues that in order for the movement to be united, it must adopt and present a coherent and consistent vegetarian ideal—an ideal that the support and promotion of ovo-lacto-vegetarianism would detract from.

The issues of defining vegetarianism and deciding how organizations should embody and express this ideology are created through ongoing negotiation processes, both within and among organizations. This process is facilitated further by the increasing use of the Internet for discussion and for information sharing. On-line comments suggest not only that some group leaders perceive that the revised definition would deter potential adherents but also that at least some groups find that they must neutralize leaders' espousal of veganism with an ideology that is more acceptable to the general public.

The Pros and Cons of an Ecumenical Ideology

National vegetarian organizations' promotion of an ecumenical ideology that embraces vegetarianism for a variety of reasons can have both positive and negative consequences. Health messages may be particularly resonant for a broad audience, for example, but vegetarians motivated by health issues may be less likely than other vegetarians to remain committed, making it difficult to sustain the movement with dedicated advocates and leaders.

Vegetarianism has a long history of intertwined ethical and health arguments, and environmental arguments are becoming an increasing area of concern. Although popular culture discourse often identifies vegetarianism as a diet of avoidances, national vegetarian organizations build upon a relatively complex ideology that provides a critique of meat-eating cultures to project the benefits of a meatless lifestyle. Organizations tend to use vegetarianism in similar ways, but there are ongoing opportunities for change, as leaders (particularly at the local level) debate how vegetarianism should be defined and local groups negotiate and formulate mission statements that reflect what they view as the ideological bases for practicing vegetarianism.

Still, changes in the vegetarian ideology are likely to be minor. Debates intended to redefine "what it means to be a vegetarian" are troublesome to movement leaders, since a broad, inclusive definition can draw the widest audience. Many leaders fear that redefining "vegetarian" too specifically—by motivation (for example, requiring that vegetarians be ethically motivated) or by rigid rules (for example, insisting that those who eat meat once a year at Thanksgiving may not call themselves vegetarians)—will prevent people from embracing vegetarianism at all.

5 The Beliefs and Strategies of Vegetarian Movement Leaders

If you eat a Twinkie, no one will listen.
—Howard Lyman, 1996 Vegetarian Summerfest

Why do movement leaders choose some strategies and overlook others? How do they determine which ones will be the most effective? Sociologists recognize several important structural factors that shape social movement strategies, including material and human resources, political constraints, and group decision-making activities,[1] but far less attention has been paid to the shared group knowledge that contributes to the strategy-making process.

In the vegetarian movement, a rich, complex set of ideas about how personal, cultural, and social changes occur channels leaders' choices about which strategies to implement and how to put them into effect. These ideas answer important questions: How do people become vegetarians? How might mainstream culture become more vegetarian friendly? How might society enact structures that support vegetarians and vegetarian diets? In general, how do changes happen, and what are the best ways to effect those changes? Although vegetarian leaders share many perspectives on these questions, most focus more on how individual people change than on how ideas and political structures and other institutions in society change.

How Do People Become Vegetarians?

Vegetarian leaders, activists, and advocates express three beliefs about how people change their diets: (1) people adopt vegetarian diets through interactions with other vegetarians; (2) although people are likely to resist dietary change initially, they may eventually embrace change; and (3) people who change their dietary practices slowly are more likely than those who change rapidly to commit to vegetarianism. These three beliefs often overlap, and a single strategy may support more than one of them. Encouraging people to gradually include more vegetarian meals in their diets supports both the belief that people initially resist dietary change and the belief that gradual change is preferable to rapid change.

Sometimes, however, a particular strategy can conflict with strategies that support other beliefs. For example, encouraging vegetarians to become ideal role models (based on the belief that social interaction helps move people toward vegetarianism) may negatively affect strategies to increase tolerance toward nonvegetarians (which are based on the belief that people are likely to resist dietary change initially). Consequently, a "perfect vegan" role model may become overly zealous and impatient with nonvegans and ultimately alienate them from vegetarianism completely.

The Importance of Social Contact

Vegetarian leaders believe that most people become vegetarians through social interaction. Although direct personal experience (such as witnessing animal slaughter or feeling disgust at the sight of raw meat) and contact with media expressions of vegetarianism (such as watching videos or reading books and magazines) may spark initial interest, social interactions enable people to interpret these experiences in support of vegetarianism. For this reason, leaders emphasize the importance of interacting with nonvegetarians. In *A Vegetarian Sourcebook*, Akers writes, "Even if it were possible for vegetarians to live a life apart from non-vegetarians, it would not be desirable; the spread of vegetarian ideas is greatly facilitated by a social mixing of vegetarians in the larger non-vegetarian population."[2] Through social interaction, vegetarian advocates can encourage others by exemplifying what it means to be a vegetarian and by giving them information about the vegetarian lifestyle. In an EarthSave International audiotape, Lyman explains, "I personally believe that survival for us is going to be one-on-one: talking to our friends, our parents, our business associates about why it is we ought to change what we're putting at the end of our fork, eating lower on the food chain, buying organic."[3] Similarly, Gary L. Francione, Rutgers University law professor and legal advisor to NAVS, told his audience at the 1995 Vegetarian Summerfest: "If you can get ten people a year to give up meat, you can do more good than most animal rights organizations."[4] Many vegetarian leaders recognize the limitations of their organizations; organizations provide outreach materials and sometimes run issue-focused campaigns, but they need individual vegetarians to inspire and motivate others.

Therefore, every vegetarian is a walking advertisement for the potential benefits and hazards of vegetarianism. The vegetarian movement strives to motivate people to change through self-interest, and positive examples can provide motivation for this change. Consequently, leaders encourage vegetarians to be physically healthy, morally consistent, and personally likable—not entirely for the benefit of practicing vegetarians but more to provide exemplars of behavior and appearance that others will want to emulate.

Encouraging vegetarians to exemplify good health is especially important in North America, where most people become vegetarians for health reasons.[5] Those ethically motivated vegetarians who are unconcerned about personal health
can detract from this positive image. At the 1995 Vegetarian
Summerfest, some lecturers extended the health emphasis to
include grooming and appearance. One speaker put it succinctly, "Learn how not to look strange," and another told audience members that when meeting with the press, they
should leave their "nose ring[s] and tie-dyed T-shirt[s] at
home."[6]

Body weight can be a sensitive topic among vegetarians,
especially vegans, who seek to counter the stereotype that
eliminating meat and other animal products from the diet
makes people (especially men) too thin, weak, and pale.[7] Although leaders' body weight is rarely, if ever, publicly discussed, people comment informally about the weight of national leaders who seem to exceed or fall short of conventional
standards. Although appearance is an important means of initially attracting new people to vegetarianism, advocates are
not encouraged to pursue conventional media-perpetuated
standards of beauty (for example, by losing or gaining weight,
becoming more muscular, or wearing fashionable clothes);
they are encouraged instead to avoid outlandish appearances
and to strive for their personal best.

Leaders also encourage vegetarians to be morally consistent and enthusiastic role models—with respect to not only
their diets but also other activities and behaviors—*without* ex-
uding fanaticism. In a local vegetarian group newsletter, a
writer admonishes her readers, "Don't give off negative vibes.
Be someone that others would want to emulate. Look good,
smile, and be confident and positive. . . . You may not notice,
but you can be sure that others are watching you. Sooner than
you think they will start asking you about your diet and why
you made your choice."[8] Physician Michael Klaper, a vegan

nutrition advocate, similarly encourages vegetarian advocates at local group meetings and national conferences. His presentations—with such titles as "Vegan Power" and "The Heart of the Matter"—often focus on exemplary action and the development of personal compassion as means of attracting new people to vegetarianism. As he told one of his audiences at the 1995 Vegetarian Summerfest, "The vegan ideal is in every human heart. Don't let anger or feelings for revenge get in the way. The only way to teach is by example. You don't have to say the "v" word; just do it. Stay gentle and respectful."[9] Leaders regard each vegetarian as having the potential to attract new adherents by socializing and setting good examples. They encourage vegetarians to strive, unbegrudgingly, for moral consistency and to be happy and positive in their efforts. They stress that being likable, friendly, warm, and open can encourage others to consider vegetarianism.

Part of the strategy of encouraging advocates to embody positive personal and moral characteristics is to ask that they remember that most vegetarians once ate meat or other animal products. At the national vegetarian and vegan conferences I attended, only one or two people in each audience of several hundred responded affirmatively when asked if anyone had been vegan since birth. Leaders encourage advocates not to become frustrated or angry with meat eaters but to empathize with them instead.

In his opening comments at the 1995 International Vegan Festival, for example, Peter McQueen, president of VUNA, told his audience, "Although we must work and strive to promote vegetarianism and veganism, we also need to be tolerant and . . . recognize that—for most of us—we were once eating meat or eating other animal products. It is only through understanding and tolerance and public education that we will draw people to a better lifestyle."[10] In a lecture entitled "Sharing Veganism in a Nonjudgmental Way," Stacey Vicari continued this theme later in the program: "The reality is that we all ate meat and/or dairy products in our lifetime, but now we 'get it.' . . . Then the reality that we ever ate that way—we forget about that. So it's really important when you deliver your tone to people that it's really inclusive. . . . If you want to invite somebody to look at your diet, be a perfect role model."[11]

Those Who Resist May Eventually Change

Vegetarian leaders generally agree that most people are extremely resistant to changing their dietary attitudes and practices but that people who are initially very resistant may eventually become interested. People often spend a lot of time thinking about meat eating and vegetarianism before they become willing to change their eating habits. Leaders emphasize the importance of spreading the vegetarian message in ways that minimize the resistance that people are likely to feel when confronted with the possibility of change. Although there is no uniform strategy among leaders for reducing prospective adherents' resistance, several leaders have noted specific ways to minimize defensiveness.

Vegetarian activist Pamela Rice of the VivaVegie Society wears a sandwich board with the words "Ask Me Why I'm a Vegetarian," as she hands out her "101 Reasons Why I'm a Vegetarian" on the streets of New York City. Her choice of titles is intended to minimize resistance: "The tactic is not to tell people that they should be a vegetarian. Many people get defensive. Even though there's nothing around me saying, '*You* should be a vegetarian' . . . people project that in their minds often. . . . I [make] it as clear as I possibly [can] that this is 101 reasons why *I'm* a vegetarian and ask me why *I'm* a vegetarian. And if you're ready to listen, I'll tell you."[12] By focusing on her own choices rather than making demands on others, Rice invites people to think about vegetarianism without the threat of having to make any immediate changes.

Strategies to reduce people's resistance to dietary change often focus on the use of nonthreatening language. In particular, many leaders—even those from the explicitly vegan organizations (AVS, Vegan Outreach, and Vegan Action)—avoid use of the word "vegan" when addressing general audiences. As one leader put it, "When you say 'vegan,' it gets [you] a blank stare," and as another explained, "The 'vegan' word scares people."[13] Just as many people did not know the meaning of "vegetarian" in the 1960s (and many people today think vegetarians eat fish), today "vegan" is a relatively unknown term; even many vegetarians are unsure about its pronunciation (vē′-gən).

When Vegan Outreach activists distribute their "Why Vegan?" brochures on college campuses, they ask people, "Would you like some information about *vegetarianism*?" According to Ball, they usually ask this because "that's a familiar word to them. And you're only going to have this interaction with them for a brief instant. So you have to catch their imagination. If you say, 'veganism,' most people are just going to say, 'Buddhism,' another weird 'ism,' and walk past. So we say 'vegetarianism' because it connects with people."[14] The idea is that most people have heard the term "vegetarianism" and that people are more likely to view a familiar term than an unfamiliar term as positive. In fact, even though many local vegetarian societies are headed by ethically motivated vegans, only one local group that completed a survey for this book uses "vegan" in its name. Since that time, a couple of new local vegan groups have adopted the word "vegan" as part of their names, but the vast majority use "vegetarian" as a means of reducing people's resistance.

At EarthSave International, advocates go a step farther. They avoid the terms "vegetarians" and "vegans," opting instead for the phrase "people who follow vegetarian [or vegan or plant-based] diets." Vicari explains, "When I say 'I'm a

vegetarian,' what [people are] hearing is not that *I'm* a vegetarian; they're hearing, 'Are *you* a vegetarian? I want to make
you a vegetarian if you're not a vegetarian.' Whereas when I
say, 'Yes, I eat a vegetarian diet,' there's a pause, a pause that
gives them the space to know I'm talking about myself and my
own preferences, not necessarily theirs.[15] The EarthSave International website (see Appendix B) presents the following
question and answer on its "frequently asked questions" page:
"Do I need to eat a vegetarian diet to join? Definitely NOT!!
EarthSave accepts you wherever you are on the food-choice
continuum. In fact, we prefer to talk about eating a more
plant-based diet and not to label anyone 'a vegetarian.'" In
other words, some leaders perceive that carefully selected language can encourage people to become more open to vegetarianism.

Other groups, in addition to EarthSave International,
adopt the term "plant-based" when they determine that a particular audience might perceive it as less threatening than
"vegetarian" or "vegan." For example, Vegan Action used the
term "plant-based" rather than "vegan" when it initiated its
campaign to encourage dining halls at the University of California at Berkeley to include a vegan option at every meal.
Vegan Action founder Leor Jacobi encourages others to take
a similar approach: "The most important factor in waging an
effective campaign is to mainstream the idea of a vegan dorm
option. . . . For example: Instead of saying 'we are advocating
a vegan diet,' it may be more effective to say 'we are advocating a more healthy, environmentally sound, plant based
diet.'"[16] Leaders often determine that their ideas may be more
acceptable to mainstream audiences if they replace the unfamiliar and potentially politically charged word "vegan" (which
some may associate with animal rights activism) with "vegetarian" or "plant-based diet."

Most vegetarian groups spread their messages through
books, pamphlets, and magazines, which are increasingly be-

coming available on the organizations' Internet web pages. In addition, leaders consider conferences—where attendees learn new information that they can share with others—as strong vehicles for spreading the idea of vegetarianism. Leaders generally believe that although most people resist dietary change, not all people resist equally. Because it is impossible to know exactly who may be drawn to the vegetarian message, some leaders advocate the strategy of spreading the vegetarian message as widely as possible without being concerned about immediate results (that is, without being concerned about converting people to vegetarianism or veganism instantaneously).

Organizers generally stress the importance of "planting seeds" through social interaction and at vegetarian conferences, but they focus on children, teenagers, and college students as the most easily influenced populations. In other words, some "soils" are more fertile than others, and these are the preferable places to plant vegetarian "seeds." For example, according to Ball, Vegan Outreach targets college students because "they're in a situation where they're able to explore new possibilities, [and] they're not living at home under their parents' roof. And they're not older and more embedded in their practices. And so, theoretically, they're in the best position to be able to change of anyone."[17] Several of the national groups target young people through their efforts to introduce vegetarianism into course curricula. In EarthSave International's *Healthy School Lunch Action Guide,* Susan Campbell and Todd Winant explain why they offer encouragement to community members who strive to bring vegetarianism into school classrooms and lunchrooms: "Students' lives are shaped by every single thing that happens. Sometimes the tiniest choice alters an entire life. . . . It might be years until an idea or sentence they've heard surfaces in their awareness. Let us nurture our youth, for they are the garden of our future."[18] Leaders hope that the information that students receive and the activities that they experience will have a future, dramatic impact. The idea that ultimately one never knows who will be affected by a vegetarian message reassures advocates that their efforts are not made in vain.

Slow Change Is Better Than Rapid Change

The belief that slow change is better than rapid change follows from the belief that those who resist may eventually change. Most vegetarian leaders hold not only that people tend to resist dietary change and that some groups are more likely to change than others but also that—for those who do change—it is best to change gradually. Perhaps this belief merely rationalizes the fact that most people become vegetarians gradually and that most ovo-lacto-vegetarians never become vegans. As Rice puts it, "I think that when most people come to vegetarianism they kind of crawl along from one stage to another."[19]

Leaders express concern that those who move too quickly from meat eating to complete veganism may become discouraged and give up all efforts to embrace vegetarianism. In *Animal Liberation,* Singer warns that if people become so overwhelmed "that they end up doing nothing at all . . . the exploitation of animals will continue as before."[20] Similarly, in a handout for a 1995 Vegetarian Summerfest presentation entitled "Starting and Running a Local Group," Binghamton, New York's Club Veg founder, Amie Hamlin, writes, "We find that encouraging people to eat more vegetarian food is much less threatening than encouraging vegetarianism. Responses to this approach are much less defensive, and probably lead to less animal product consumption overall. Once defensiveness is gone, and health benefits are felt, there is a greater chance of people 'going all the way'—becoming vegetarian." Vegetarian advocates also want to encourage people to feel good about whatever changes they do make. For example, Judy Krizmanic, author of *A Teen's Guide to Going Vegetarian,* tells her readers, "Take things at your own pace, and as far as *you* want to take them. If you want to stop eating red meat, and that's all, then just stop eating red meat. Maybe you'll eventually stop eating other meat, too, but don't get caught up in a guilt trip if you don't. Celebrate that you have successfully given up red meat. That's something!"[21] Focusing on the positive aspects of gradual change downplays vegetarianism's "absoluteness" and encourages people to view the change as a series of choices, a set of alternatives. If people perceive that the only way to "go vegetarian" is to forgo all meat products (or in the case of veganism, all animal products) immediately, they may resist change altogether. Vegetarian leaders try to minimize the negative connotations of vegetarianism (such as restriction and rigidity) and create a more positive impression of the vegetarian lifestyle. They do so by encouraging vegetarian advocates—as exemplary role models—to delight in whatever dietary changes people make toward vegetarianism and to offer gentle, positive, and subtle encouragement of future changes.

Most, though not all, vegetarian (and even vegan) advocates view gradual change as positive. Two physicians who promote vegetarianism, Dean Ornish and Neil Barnard, both advocate rapid, drastic changes in diet.[22] They hold that when people switch directly to vegan or near-vegan diets, they often experience a dramatic improvement that motivates them to adhere to a vegetarian diet. According to Ornish:

> What we have found, paradoxically, is that big changes are easier than small ones, because you feel so much better. Conventional wisdom is that small, gradual changes are easy, and big, rapid changes are hard. . . . But when you make moderate changes, you get the worst of both worlds. You feel deprived because you're not getting to eat and do everything that you enjoy, but you're not making changes big enough to get much benefit. . . . When people make comprehensive changes, they begin to feel so much better that they find that the changes are worth making.[23]

Vegetarian leaders often cite the work of Ornish and Barnard and quote the authors in their groups' publications; to date, however, organization leaders have not adopted the notion of promoting rapid dietary change.

How Might Mainstream Culture Become More Vegetarian Friendly?

Because most people become vegetarians out of concern for their personal health rather than out of political consciousness, the vegetarian movement—while it *aspires* to cultural, and in some cases, social changes—focuses primarily on changing individuals and to a lesser degree on educating converted vegetarians about the ethical reasons for vegetarianism. The social and cultural changes that organizations pursue (such as making vegetarian foods available in fast-food restaurants and changing federal School Lunch Program guidelines to include vegetarian alternatives) are typically those that movement leaders believe will lead more individuals to adopt vegetarian diets.

Most organizations *aspire to* broad-based cultural changes that would bring about a "vegetarian world"; however, ultimately, most vegetarian advocates view these changes as being most likely to occur one person at a time. Vegetarian leaders, activists, and advocates express two basic beliefs about cultural change: (1) Cultural changes require that people recognize that eating animal products is a cultural tradition rather than a biological necessity. (2) Cultural changes occur because of individual and collective demands and market responses to those demands.

Cultural Changes Require Lifting "The Meat Spell"

A basic vegetarian assumption is that meat is not only unnecessary for but also deleterious to human health and well-being.

Culture, not nature, motivates and perpetuates meat consumption. Karen Iacobbo and Michael Gibson have dubbed this hold that culture has on people "the meat spell": "'The meat spell' is our term for the belief that meat is a necessary and appetizing part of the human diet. Why a spell? Because the belief is usually based upon 'facts,' tradition or habits the meat-eater hasn't challenged."[24] "The meat spell," say Iacobbo and Gibson, must be lifted in order for vegetarianism to become culturally valued and accepted.

Some vegetarians argue that meat eating is not only the product of a cultural "spell" but also an *unnatural* practice. They present a biological rationale for vegetarianism, arguing that human physiology is closest to that of the herbivores, who by nature eat a vegan diet. In a local vegetarian group newsletter, a writer asks, "Do you believe that meat will make you strong and healthy? Then you have bought into a commercial propaganda myth. In truth, human beings are neither carnivores (meat eater) nor omnivorous (meat and grain) but strictly herbivorous (grains, herbs, fruits & vegetables)."[25] Vegetarian leaders point out that meat eaters avoid the guilt associated with killing animals for food with such mechanisms as cooking meat in sauces and using the terms "pork" and "beef" rather than "pig" and "cow." This, they suggest, supports their view that humans are not meant to consume meat.[26] Iacobbo and Gibson write, "Some people say that humans are omnivores, or designed to consume plants and animals. But natural omnivores don't have to hide the fact that they are eating dead animals from themselves. Only people do that. True meat-eaters don't have to cook flesh or disguise it with salt, ketchup, and a slice of onion."[27] Similarly, Klaper tells his readers, "Humans are not carnivorous by their anatomy, nor by their nature. If we were true carnivores, we would walk into a butcher shop, purchase a large slab of raw cow flesh, leave the store, sit down on the curb, tear off the wrapping paper, and devour the bloody flesh with gusto."[28]

Many vegetarian leaders view veganism as the most natural human diet and meat eating as an unnatural cultural phenomenon that many people will abandon once they are exposed to the vegetarian message in a positive way.

Arguing that a totally vegetarian (completely herbivorous—that is, vegan) diet is the most natural diet for humans can be strategically problematic, however. Unlike an ovolacto-vegetarian diet, which can meet all nutritional requirements without supplementation, a vegan diet lacks one essential nutrient: vitamin B_{12}. Today B_{12} is found naturally only in meat, dairy products, and eggs; it is produced by bacteria in the digestive tracts of animals. B_{12} deficiencies, though quite rare, can cause serious damage to the nervous system. This nutritional inadequacy is problematic for those who promote veganism, particularly for those who promote veganism as the most natural human diet. B_{12} has even been called the "Achilles heel" of veganism.[29] According to Akers:

> The only real issue I see that is outstanding against veganism is B_{12}. Which is an extremely serious issue in terms of the public promulgation of veganism, but is not an internal issue. The response is, for people in the movement, "B_{12}. No problem. Take a tablet. . . ." But [not so] for an outsider who says, "So, you're telling me that this diet *lacks* an essential nutrient? And you want the entire country to be put on this diet? So you want me to take a vitamin supplement. . . . Why am I taking vitamin supplements if this diet is supposed to be so healthy?"[30]

One way to neutralize the accusation that vegan diets are unnatural because they lack a "natural" source of B_{12} is to argue that it is actually our "unnatural" food production processes that inhibit the availability of B_{12} in plant-based foods. According to Klaper, "Fresh garden vegetables, with microscopic soil particles clinging to them that contain Vitamin B-12, as well as foods fermented in porcelain vats, like tempeh and miso, were traditionally rich sources of Vitamin B-12. Now, however, due to industrial production of vegetables, and to sanitation of stainless steel fermenting vats, these food products can no longer be relied upon as adequate B-12 sources."[31] Arguments about the unnatural nature of meat consumption often assert that in a perfect state of nature, all the nutritional needs of a vegan would be met.

Other advocates present the view that although humans are not biologically *incapable* of meat eating, they are best suited to vegetarian diets. Those who take this position stress that social, moral, and health arguments are more apt to encourage vegetarianism than are arguments that emphasize biological reductionism. According to an NAVS brochure entitled "Vegetarianism: Answers to the Most Commonly Asked Questions":

> Animals closest to us physiologically are vegetarian or nearly vegetarian, and so were our not too distant evolutionary ancestors. . . . While scientists disagree about specific anatomy and physiology points, one of the best indications that humans are best suited to a vegetarian diet is the many benefits found with plant-based diets and the many diseases and illnesses linked to eating meat. The ability to eat an omnivorous diet may have had survival value in the past but it is now clear that meat-eating threatens human health and planetary survival.

One way to encourage cultural acceptance of vegetarianism (and to lift "the meat spell") has been to highlight mainstream studies whose findings support the healthfulness of vegetarian diets. When vegetarian publications cast vegetarian diets as optimally healthful and diets that include meat as hazardous to the health, they often use conventional scientific research to back their claims.[32] As one vegetarian author put it, "Vegetarianism, once it has achieved a solid scientific foundation, will become the 'norm' in Western nations."[33] Groups often cite positive statements about vegetarian diets made by the ADA and the USDA. When the USDA proclaimed vegetarian diets to be healthful, for example, FARM sent out its 1996 Meat-Out fund-raising letter in an envelope reading, "USDA

Endorses Meat-Out Pledge." Even such authors as Jon Wynne-Tyson, who argue on moral and ecological grounds, claim that the health arguments for vegetarianism should be presented first, in order to counteract the mainstream cultural acceptance of meat as a healthful and desirable food.[34]

Another strategy for lifting "the meat spell" is to highlight weaknesses in meat-eating culture as they arise, particularly in the popular media. For example, believing that the popularity of the movie *Babe* reveals a crack in meat-eating culture, in several cities, vegetarian groups handed out leaflets with veg-etarian information as patrons left theaters after seeing the movie. In the film, Babe, an affable pig, demonstrates his value and intelligence by learning to herd sheep. He is partic-ularly motivated to prove his worth after learning that humans consumed his parents and that, ultimately, he will suffer the same fate. As a promotional tie-in with the movie, McDon-ald's began to offer *Babe* toys with its Happy Meals, advertis-ing the promotion on national television with the exhortation "Buy one, and your kids can pretend they're Babe."[35] As a re-sult of this promotion, some activists distributed a Farm Sanc-tuary flyer called "Babe's *Unhappy* Meal": "Like Babe in the movie, all animals have feelings—including the pigs, cows, and chickens who were raised and slaughtered for McDon-ald's menu. Babe didn't want to be killed to become some-one's 'meal,' and neither do the billions of farm animals now suffering at slaughterhouses across the country. Babe knows the only 'happy meal' is a 'veggie' meal, and he needs your help to encourage McDonald's to serve a vegetarian burger." Other groups adopted the Babe icon as well. Members of the VivaVegie Society in New York City carried a three-foot-tall cardboard cutout of Babe as they leafleted the sausage ven-dors at the Feast of San Gennero. According to the group's newsletter, "Between the ears of the endearing portrait of our intrepid hero 'Babe,' VivaVegie placed the simple statement, 'Sausage Kills Me.' And these words combined with the lovable image of 'Babe' made quite a sensation."[36] In 1997, PETA used the Babe image in a protest at the North Carolina Pork Producers Association's annual conference in Fayetteville, North Carolina. On a highway overpass during the morning rush hour, a PETA activist dressed as Babe unfurled a banner reading "Meat is Murder." (An account of this protest can be found on PETA's website [see Appendix B].) PETA also distributes a "Please Don't Eat Babe for Breakfast" poster.

National-level journalists have also used Babe as an icon that represents how the public thinks about farm animals. Recent concerns about the odor that emanates from large-scale hog farms—particularly in North Carolina—has brought farm conditions to the public's attention as an environmental, rather than an animal rights, issue. Reporters note the disparity between the life of Babe in the film and the life of a typical pig on a factory farm. After some video footage made this contrast in a 1996 segment called "Pork Power" on *60 Minutes,* journalist Morley Safer commented:

> This [video footage from the film *Babe*] is more like the way Americans want to think of pigs. . . . Real-life "Babes" see no sun in their limited lives with no hay to lie on, no mud to roll in and do not talk. The sows live in tiny cages, so narrow they can't even turn around. They live over metal grates, and their waste is pushed through slats beneath them and flushed into huge pits. It's the waste that's the problem. . . . It's turning North Carolina into one vast toilet.[37]

A *Washington Post* article strengthened the connection between *Babe,* hog farms, and vegetarianism, by quoting from a letter about the hog odor problem written by James Cromwell—identified as a vegan who portrayed Farmer Hoggett in *Babe*—to North Carolina's governor, James Hunt. The article also quotes a representative of PETA as saying, "As long as people eat meat, there will be odor."[38]

Vegetarian publications celebrate these popular culture manifestations of vegetarianism. Lisa Simpson—the animated, socially conscious daughter on "The Simpsons," who became a vegetarian on the show in 1995—is another celebrated vegetarian icon. Celebrities, such as Mary Tyler Moore, Woody Harrelson, Paul and Linda McCartney, and Chrissie Hynde (of the rock group the Pretenders)—who often mention and discuss their vegetarianism in media interviews—are also honored. Vegetarian leaders interpret the increasing amount of celebrity publicity and the growing number of vegetarian characters on television (including Phoebe on "Friends" and Darlene on "Roseanne") as further evidence that vegetarianism is becoming more mainstream and that "the meat spell" can be broken.

The Importance of Individual and Collective Demands

Vegetarian leaders hold that because companies act in their own financial interest, cultural changes are possible when vegetarians make their wishes and demands known to producers and retailers. If businesses think they can make money by producing vegetarian products, they are likely to do so. Vegetarian leaders greatly value these cultural changes because the availability of vegetarian foods is key to attracting new vegetarians and keeping present ones committed. The importance of social interaction and access to positive information about vegetarianism in encouraging vegetarianism suggests that a culture amenable to vegetarianism would facilitate this process. As Ball explains, "You have three stages: when people become aware of things, and then, when a small portion of the people change because they're really converted, and finally, it becomes easy. So people have said, 'If it was easy to be a vegetarian, I'd be a vegetarian.'"[39] Current improvements in the availability of vegetarian foods suggest that placing demands on the consumer market can successfully effect retailer compliance.

A primary strategy for vegetarian organizations—based on the idea that cultural changes are possible when people demand them and economic consequences are at stake—is to encourage people to ask local restaurants, fast-food chains, and other businesses to offer vegetarian products. The NAVS Vegetarian Express: Fast Food Campaign, for example, encourages people to call fast-food retailers, request that they provide plant-based entrées, and then send copies of any correspondence back to NAVS. An NAVS brochure promoting the campaign states:

> NAVS believes strongly that fast food restaurants—like all other businesses—want to cater to consumer demands. Quite simply, if enough people ask for vegetarian alternatives at fast food restaurants, we will undoubtedly get them. It's that simple. So what NAVS is doing is organizing the consumer demand and monitoring the results. We will continue to inform officials at fast food corporations that there is a growing market for plant-based entrées.

As part of this campaign, NAVS also tries to secure from fast-food retailers lists of the vegan products that they offer on their menus. In most cases, the options are few; for example, at McDonald's, the vegan menu is limited to various sauces and toppings, salads, and breakfast cereals; at Domino's Pizza, since the pizza crusts contain some animal-derived ingredients, only the sauce is vegan.

Similarly, Vegan Action and Farm Sanctuary conduct campaigns to encourage fast-food retailers to include vegetarian options. In March 1996, Vegan Action began a McVegan campaign, which encourages people to sign its petition requesting that McDonald's "add a healthy and tasty, cholesterol-free vegan burger to its menu as a new option." Farm Sanctuary has encouraged people to lobby for a vegetarian option at McDonald's, and, according to *Sanctuary News,* the group's newsletter, the organization "prompted Burger King [in Watkins Glen, New York] to introduce the first fast-food vegetarian burger."[40]

As vegetarian organizations lobby fast-food chains such as McDonald's, Burger King, and Subway to offer vegetarian items, some individual vegetarians debate whether it is morally acceptable at all to eat at fast-food chains that also serve meat products. Should one support a business that contributes to animal suffering and death? Vegetarian organizations take the view that each new vegetarian entrée that appears on the menu of a mainstream fast-food restaurant chain constitutes a small victory.

The controversy over whether to frequent fast-food chains has attracted increasing attention, with the 1995 London trial of environmental activists Dave Morris and Helen Steel, who were charged with libelous actions against the McDonald's corporation for handing out a six-page leaflet entitled "What's Wrong with McDonald's? Everything They Don't Want You to Know."[41] According to a *Washington Post* article, the leaflet contains allegations "that McDonald's food isn't nutritious because of its high fat content, that the company has forced employees under age 18 to work longer than the law allows and that its meat comes from cattle who graze in areas that used to be rainforests."[42] Because in England, the defendant must prove that allegedly libelous material is true (whereas in the United States, the plaintiff must prove that the allegations are false), the "McLibel" trial (as it has come to be known) continued in London's Royal Courts of Justice for more than two and a half years. The activists deliberately dragged out the trial and used the courtroom as a venue for the presentation of a wide range of evidence—including testimonies from vegan advocates Lyman and Barnard—to back their claims and to generate publicity against McDonald's. Ultimately, the defendants lost the case and were admonished to pay Mc-

Donald's sixty thousand pounds in damages; upon appeal, in January and February 1999, the court reduced the damages but did not overturn the verdict.

The trial has resulted in many protests against McDonald's internationally, centering on World Anti-McDonald's Day, the October 16 day of action started by London Greenpeace in the mid-1980s. Most of these protests are spearheaded by animal rights rather than vegetarian organizations (with the exception of the VivaVegie Society, a local, activist-oriented vegetarian group in New York City), and many of these direct actions result in news coverage and arrests. In California, for example, "activists from Santa Cruz Animal Rights (SCAR) and the Bay Area Animal Rights Direct Action Coalition (BAARDAC) locked themselves to chairs and tables with kryptonite locks. Despite taunts from customers, who shoved Big Macs in their faces, the activists stayed. Police later ejected and arrested three of the activists, and dragged one of them out by her hair."[43] And in Minneapolis:

> there were four arrests when activists from SOAR (Student Organization for Animal Rights) took over the roof of a McDonald's for about two hours. They used the "human octopus"—where people bikelock themselves together—to frustrate police. . . . Activists were maced and sent to the hospital, spending five hours in "detox" before being moved to jail and charged with trespassing. . . . There was substantial news coverage, including television, radio, and print.[44]

These direct actions by animal rights groups contrast markedly with vegetarian groups' efforts to request more vegetarian options. Whereas vegetarian groups typically stress polite behavior and express appreciation for even minor changes in a positive direction, animal rights groups are more likely to engage in acts of civil disobedience that offend some people, cause chaos, and bring public attention to an issue. Whereas animal rights groups tend to emphasize conflict with a known enemy (for example, McDonald's or a scientist who conducts laboratory experiments with animals), vegetarian groups, in their efforts to effect cultural change, focus on consensual solutions: win-win situations in which vegetarians gain more dietary options and retailers make more money.

At the local level, too, vegetarian groups try to initiate cultural change in a nonconflictual manner, by requesting that local (not necessarily fast-food) restaurants and grocery stores offer more vegetarian foods. For example, when a new grocery store was set to open in Toledo, Ohio, members of the local vegetarian society called the store's corporate staff to encourage them to include a vegetarian/health food section in their food court.[45] Although sometimes group members ask restaurant and store owners directly, they usually use more subtle techniques. Many local groups, for example, sponsor weekly or monthly dinner outings at restaurants, some of which already have a vegetarian orientation but many of which are just becoming interested in offering vegetarian cuisine. The Vegetarian Club of Canton (VCC) portrays these outings as opportunities to encourage positive cultural change. As a 1995 VCC "Calendar and Information Brochure" explains, "Through the monthly dinner program, the VCC is paying for the area restaurant owners, food service managers, chefs, waiters, and waitresses to take the time to learn how to cook and serve quality vegetarian meals. Our hope is that over time many of these meals will end up on the menus of these establishments. This has already begun to happen." Like the national organizations, local groups recognize that an economic incentive encourages retailers to change.

Vegetarians sometimes even extend these incentives to restaurant staff. In the article "Rethinking Restaurant Tipping," which is available on VRG's website (see Appendix B), Carole Hamlin argues that vegetarians should always tip a higher percentage of their bills than meat eaters. Otherwise, since vegetarian meals cost less than meat-centered meals, staff may be less attentive to vegetarians because they may assume they will not benefit financially from their patronage. Hamlin explains, "I want to encourage restaurants to offer vegetarians options without having to fight the waiters." Similarly, the Vegetarian Society of El Paso's 1994 brochure "Vegetarian Dining Guide for El Paso" encourages vegetarians to create positive interactions with restaurant staff: "You may be surprised at how accommodating restaurant staff can be if you take a positive attitude and make them your partners in satisfying your dietary needs, rather than being contrary, contentious or apologetic. . . . Keep in mind that our primary mission is to educate people. Leave your waiter or waitress with the information and a positive experience to provide better service for the next vegetarian." Local group strategies for cultural change focus on seeking more vegetarian options within their communities. Like the national groups, they concentrate on providing retailers with economic incentives for including vegetarian items and generating a positive, nonconflictual image of the typical vegetarian. Local and national vegetarian organizations (unlike animal rights organizations) typically do not challenge the fast-food industry's commitment to selling meat; instead, they encourage retailers to offer more vegetarian alternatives to fast-food meat items.

How Might Social Structures Change to Benefit Vegetarian Movement Goals?

Although in the vegetarian movement talk of structural change may be increasing, it is still fairly uncommon. Leaders rarely publicly discuss strategies for enhancing the power of vegetarians as a group or for making concrete legislative changes that promote or support vegetarianism. Even rarer are discussions of *how* such concrete structural changes could occur.

The only national vegetarian organization to articulate how *institutional* changes are likely to occur is VRG, which is concerned with effecting changes in schools, hospitals, and public assistance programs. In this group's view, educating people in power is the most effective way to promote social change. As co-founder Debra Wasserman explains, "In our society in order to make change, you have to influence these people who are in power, whether it be locally or nationally, or internationally. And so our focus and interest is reaching that level because the only way you're really going to make change . . . is you have to set up an infrastructure to make that change possible."[46] VRG employs dietitians to speak about vegetarian issues to professional audiences and to participate in policy decisions with respect to programs such as the National Meals on Wheels Foundation (with which it created a vegetarian menu plan for seniors) and the federal School Lunch Program.[47] The dietitians also create vegetarian publications, which VRG distributes on request to individuals, schools, and other organizations. In addition, VRG staffs booths at professional meetings of the AHA, the American School Food Service Association, the ADA, and other groups and puts out the publication *Food Service Update*, which includes information and large-quantity recipes for hospitals, schools, and other large institutions.

Unlike other organizations that focus on promoting vegetarianism at the individual level, VRG seeks to influence those in power to change rules so that vegetarian foods become more available and accepted in institutions. VRG has also indirectly influenced the ADA. As Suzanne Havala, nutrition advisor to VRG, explains, material from VRG publications (much of which she wrote) has ultimately been co-opted by the ADA:

> It's taken several years, but by and large, what's available out there as a resource in the way of vegetarian nutrition materials comes from the VRG. . . . ADA's publishing a book, a big general book on nutrition, and they sent me the authors' vegetarian chapter to [review]. And I could literally follow the VRG materi-

als straight through the chapter. I could have told you each
brochure and each hand-out that the person got the material
from. So I thought to myself, "Wow, the VRG most decidedly
has had a big influence on dietitians."[48]

VRG influences the nutrition profession by hiring professional
dietitians to produce materials that use appropriate scientific
language and jargon and to research data from professionally
legitimate scientific publications; VRG then promotes these
materials in an institutionally acceptable way. More than any
other vegetarian organization, VRG is concerned with effecting change by legitimizing vegetarianism in centers of power.

Other organizations occasionally suggest the potential
benefits of social change, but these efforts are rare and, for the
most part, have not progressed much beyond the discussion
stage. The VivaVegie Society in New York City is initiating a
Project for Economic Justice for Vegetarians, which focuses
on documenting how the U.S. government subsidizes meat
production and consumption. A VivaVegie flyer describes the
ultimate goal of the project as "not to antagonize, but to call
attention to the injustice of meat sponsorship either bla-
tantly—by hard core dollar subsidies and tax breaks from federal and local governments, or through ignorance or habit—
by doctors, insurance companies, educators, commercial
entities and the like." The flyer argues that those who consume animal products should pay for the government costs of
its production, and it asks that federal meat subsidies be
ended. In the VivaVegie Society group newsletter, a group
member adds that vegetarians should get a tax deduction and
that "perhaps vegetarians should sue the government in a
class-action suit for unfair taxation, or withhold a percentage
of their taxes as promoted by the War Resisters League."[49]

Taking a slightly different direction, some individuals and
groups have begun to make legal claims for vegetarianism,
and there is some indication that vegetarian groups may become involved in future legal battles. For example, in 1996,

California bus driver Bruce Anderson filed a lawsuit against the Orange County Transportation Authority, after he was dismissed for refusing to hand out free hamburger coupons for a local fast-food restaurant.[50] The U.S. Equal Opportunity Commission ruled in Anderson's favor, stating that his employer violated laws against religious discrimination and that Anderson held his vegetarian beliefs with the same conviction that many others hold traditional religious views.

Recently, other individuals and groups have sued or have begun plans to sue fast-food companies (including Wendy's and McDonald's) for misrepresenting foods that contain some animal ingredients as vegetarian or all vegetable. One such organization is the Vegetarian Legal Awareness Network (VLAN), which was founded in 1999 by six law students "to establish and defend the rights of vegetarians."[51] VLAN has petitioned the U.S. Food and Drug Administration (FDA) to require that food manufacturers identify on their product labels the many ingredients (some of which are animal derived) that are now called "natural flavors."

Because vegetarian groups typically do not see the evolution of a vegetarian world occurring through legal changes, most avoid provoking conflict and resolving grievances through litigation. If VLAN's efforts receive adequate publicity, however, they will probably generate new dialogue among vegetarian advocates about how social change occurs.

Changing Culture and Society One Person at a Time

Although most leaders argue that it is *possible* to effect broader social and, especially, cultural change and believe that they are working toward achieving that goal, many stress the primary importance of *individual* action and change. Although the vegetarian movement as a whole promotes some cultural and social changes, *fundamentally* it relies on personal change in order to effect movement goals. According to a 1996 Vegan

Outreach brochure, "*Fundamental change* will come one person at a time, as awareness and understanding grows [*sic*] and attitudes and outlook are expanded."[52] Vegan Action Executive Director David Blatte echoes this perspective: "Personal contact is what we are about. The world will not change all at once. It will change one person at a time."[53] So as organizations attempt to effect broad changes such as those described herein, leaders—who view individual actions as a means of reducing animal suffering and spreading the vegetarian message—continue to emphasize the importance of *changing people*. For example, Dinshah writes, "To change the appalling conditions that exist for the animals requires changes in our lifestyles. Reform depends on our individual actions, on the choices we make everyday [*sic*]."[54] The primary, overarching strategy, then, is not to effect change through collective action but to change the world through collective individual improvement. As each vegetarian becomes more grounded in the vegetarian ethic, he or she is expected to become an increasingly powerful resource for attracting and motivating others. In *The Most Noble Diet,* George Eisman, founder of the vegetarian nutrition organization VEGEDINE, writes, "By living a more Noble life, we can experience the joy of knowing we are doing our part in building a better world, a better community, a better environment, and a better self. . . . Only when we choose to shape our own destinies, by solving our problems by changing our behavior, can we ensure everlasting freedom for all."[55] Each vegetarian, then, is an important resource to the movement; every person's abstinence from eating meat is perceived as contributing to the movement's goal of saving animals' lives.

The vegetarian movement focuses on personal changes in diet and ethics to effect movement goals, and changing individuals' hearts and minds and especially their lifestyles and behaviors is considered key to broader cultural and social changes. Although the focus is individual change, the vegetarian movement adopts models of the ways that cultural changes are likely to occur because cultural changes facilitate the process of becoming a vegetarian. Even though leaders and groups want, and in some cases, *expect* to see a vegetarian world evolve, they rarely focus on achieving these goals by effecting structural change. Some would argue that because the movement currently lacks the resources to make such demands as tax breaks and lower insurance premiums for vegetarians, such efforts would be difficult to implement.

6 Organizational Strategy in Action

Promoting a Vegetarian Collective Identity

We want a vegan world, not a vegan club.
—Matt Ball, Jack Norris, and Anne Green, "Tips for Spreading Veganism"

To varying degrees, vegetarian leaders and their respective organizations adopt an inclusive approach to promoting vegetarianism that embraces as positive all movement toward vegetarian diets. For example, even though less than one-third of the twelve million U.S. adults who self-identify as vegetarians actually follow a vegetarian diet,[1] leaders applaud the number because they see it as evidence that many people *want* to be and like to think of themselves as vegetarians. Vegetarians also celebrate the fact that cultural stereotypes that associated their lifestyle with the hippie counterculture and youthful rebellion have given way to a general view of vegetarian diets as healthful and acceptable.

At the same time, the possible dilution of vegetarianism concerns leaders who want to protect the definition of the term from becoming meaningless. As one local group newsletter author warns, "While the actual number of vegetarians is probably lower than we may have thought, acceptance of vegetarianism and a desire to identify with it is definitely on

117

the increase, a trend that will surely benefit all of us. On the other hand, perhaps we need to get just a little possessive about the term 'vegetarian' and its definition, lest it cease to have any meaning."[2] Many vegetarians express concern that the public perceives them as people who do not eat red meat or who eat meat only occasionally. This can have a personal effect when, for example, a well-meaning host or restaurant server offers a chicken or seafood dish as a "vegetarian" alternative. Accepting a vague vegetarian definition can be not only disheartening (and perhaps even insulting) to the committed vegetarian but also potentially damaging to movement organizations, which depend on a strong identity to attract active members.

Although a nonthreatening, nonconfrontational tone may encourage people to move toward gradual adoption of vegetarian diets, inclusive movement messages that embrace all efforts toward practicing vegetarianism can dilute the vegetarian identity. And if fewer people identify strongly with organizations, fewer will be willing to volunteer and assume leadership positions. At present, less than 1 percent of the people who follow vegetarian diets belong to vegetarian groups, and far fewer are *active* members. To build their membership, organizations try to mobilize currently inactive vegetarians by educating them about the various arguments for vegetarianism; this information not only helps vegetarians articulate more solid justifications for their own practices but also provides them with a repertoire of knowledge for promoting vegetarianism to others.

Vegetarian organizations have two distinct audiences for their messages: (1) a large number of potential newcomers who are interested in vegetarian lifestyles and (2) a much smaller number of practicing vegetarians who want to learn more and who may become active advocates for vegetarianism. These two groups have very different needs and interests. The potential newcomers want to learn about the health aspects of vegetarianism, particularly about cooking with vegetarian ingredients. The practicing vegetarians want to learn more about the vegetarian philosophy or bring vegetarianism to their families, friends, and communities. The idea of having to "become a vegetarian" may repel the newcomers, many of whom may be vaguely interested in eating more vegetarian meals. The practicing vegetarians, however, need to strengthen their vegetarian identity in order to feel committed enough to contribute to movement activities.

Consequently, current leaders are very concerned with how to promote a vegetarian identity and to whom they should promote it. Leaders pose these questions: Is it more beneficial for reaching movement goals to promote a strictly "vegetarian" identity or vague "healthful, plant-based lifestyles"? Does appealing to one audience detract from appealing to another? And if so, how can both groups be reached with limited resources?

The Vegetarian Collective Identity

What does it mean to be a vegetarian? This is a key question for vegetarian organizations in developing a collective identity, "the (often implicitly) agreed upon definition of membership, boundaries, and activities for the group."[3] One particularly beneficial aspect of collective identity is that the more a person identifies with a group, the more he or she feels bound by its expectations. A committed vegetarian, for example, may feel guilty about even thinking about eating meat or ill upon unintentionally ingesting it. And a person who adopts a vegetarian identity may become increasingly aware of his or her potential role in promoting group interests. Sharing a collective sense of who they are helps motivate people to act on their beliefs.

Most movements build collective identity upon the foundation of a shared social status, such as ethnicity, gender, sexual preference, or social class. With an established collective identity, movements put potential adherents in touch with status-based traits that they already share. Various "rights" movements, for example, have mobilized people based on ethnicity, gender, and sexual preference. A collective identity magnifies a group's particular shared trait and its associated characteristics so that members come to regard the trait as central to their personal identities.

Because most people *choose* vegetarianism, however, vegetarian collective identity is different; for most (those for whom it is not a religious mandate), it is not a preexisting status but a lifestyle. As a group, vegetarians share little in common other than what they do not eat (and even that varies widely); even their motivations differ. As a result, practicing vegetarians may not readily perceive an advantage in identifying as part of a group or movement.

In addition, unlike status-based collective identities, the vegetarian collective identity does not identify any particular opponent or enemy. In other words, although the collective identify defines who "we" are (those who do not eat meat, poultry, or seafood and sometimes other animal products), it avoids defining who "they" are. Meat eaters are obvious potential "adversaries" of vegetarians, but because they are the pool of potential members, vegetarians do not want to cast them as "adversaries." Vegetarian leaders try to avoid the oppositional language of "us versus them," in favor of an approach that focuses on promoting their own activities in a positive way. For example, a Vegan Action newsletter article states:

> It is important that we always keep our message positive. The last thing in the world we need to do is to give people the impression that we're preaching to them. We can avoid this pitfall by focusing on *helping* animals, acting in *support* of the environment, *advocating* the availability of healthy foods, *promoting* veganism. In other words, being "for" something, not just against

something; being proactive, not reactive; spreading veganism, not wasting energy fighting meat-eaters.[4]

As this approach suggests, vegetarians do not want to alienate their potential audiences as they promote their collective identity. They want to be viewed as positive—in terms of what they do (supporting vegetarian causes) rather than in terms of what they *don't* do (not eating meat).

Developing the vegetarian collective identity is problematic, then, for two reasons: First, since the movement is not status-based, it does not have a pool of potential adherents with a common preexisting trait and related political interests. Second, although a vegetarian collective identity can create a sense of commonality and shared interests among vegetarians, if it becomes too strong (to the point where meat eaters become "adversaries"), vegetarian advocates risk alienating their pool of potential members. This results in a sort of balancing act, in which vegetarian organizations work both to cultivate a wide audience and to nurture the commitment of those who already practice vegetarianism.

Developing Collective Identity among Vegetarians

The people who most strongly possess a vegetarian collective identity—those committed to movement participation—tend to hold multiple reasons for their lifestyle. Though many were initially motivated by personal health benefits, over time they have come to adopt additional, ethical reasons for wanting to act on their beliefs. Aware that this is the most common scenario, many vegetarian leaders seek to move health-motivated, self-interested "exemplary" vegetarians to a more ethical focus that centers on caring more about other humans and animals. This deepening of motivation they see as being key to sparking a greater interest in vegetarian advocacy.

Most of the time and energy that vegetarian organizations expend in the development of collective identity is directed toward regional, national, and international conferences. Vegetarian organizations in the United States and Canada usually sponsor two or three large conferences annually, including the five-day Vegetarian Summerfest, the eight-day International Vegan Festival, and the World Vegetarian Congress. Some local organizations sponsor one-day regional conferences, such as the New England Vegetarian Conference. These conferences, which differ from the vegetarian food fairs and festivals that many organizations hold in order to generate the general public's interest, target an exclusive audience: people who already have an interest in, and—in most cases already practice—vegetarianism and who want to learn more about it.[5]

At these regional and national conferences, participants attend seminars, workshops, and cooking demonstrations; organizers arrange the programs so that every possible motivation (including health, animal rights, spirituality, and environment) is addressed. Because vegetarian conferences focus on those who already practice or have a strong interest in vegetarianism, the messages directed toward this exclusive audience differ from the more inclusive, general messages directed toward the general public. Conference experiences deepen and round out people's knowledge of vegetarian practices and ideology and consequently help strengthen their commitment to the movement. Conferences can lead people to espouse new reasons for their vegetarianism or help them articulate the reasons that they did not quite know how to explain before.

Because vegetarian conferences bring together those likely to become more deeply involved in the vegetarian cause, they may increase the likelihood that more of these people will move into active participation. Many leaders date their involvement with organizational activities or their commitment to following a vegan diet to their participation in a national conference. Regional and national conferences help vegetarians to articulate why they do what they do and to generate a common bond with others who share their lifestyle.

Participants at these conferences are encouraged to move from an ovo-lacto-vegetarian diet to a vegan diet. Because vegans are viewed as most committed to the movement, leaders of both the vegetarian and the animal rights movements are expected to follow a vegan diet and lifestyle. Conference lectures and workshops and organizational publications focus on both the health consequences and animal rights implications of consuming eggs and dairy products, and the conferences are successful in moving many people toward the vegan end of the vegetarian-vegan continuum. One local group leader, who started as an ovo-lacto-vegetarian for health reasons, for example, left his first Vegetarian Summerfest, in 1994, as a vegan concerned with animal rights; he estimated that, as a result of the lectures and discussions, one-third of the ovo-lacto-vegetarians that he met at the conference switched to a vegan diet.

Regional and national conferences also provide an environment for networking and offer sessions about how to organize for the movement; they are "training camps" for vegetarian advocacy and activism. The 1999 Vegetarian Summerfest, for example, sponsored a series of workshops entitled "Community Outreach: Making a Difference," which included sessions such as "Local Vegetarian Groups: Starting One and Keeping It Alive," "How Do We Get the Public to Listen? Panelists Share Their Tips and Experiences," and "Spreading the Vegetarian Message in Small Town USA." Some participants use the information they collect at conference lectures to enhance local group activities. Attendees meet others with similar interests, make new friends, and develop social networks that may motivate them to participate more actively in movement organizations.

Many people, especially those who live in relatively isolated, nonurban areas, find that attending a conference with four hundred or five hundred other vegetarians is a very powerful, energizing, and friendship-building experience. Even so, only a small percentage of vegetarians attends these conferences. This may be explained in part by the financial costs of attendance; the fee for the five-day Vegetarian Summerfest, for example, is $527 for a single adult, which does not including transportation to the conference site, and although children are welcome, the cost for a family can be prohibitive. This strategy for building collective identity, as a result, reaches a limited audience of potential leaders.

Collective Identity: An Asset or Liability for Attracting New Vegetarians?

As we have noted, although a strong collective identity can encourage current vegetarians to become more involved in movement activities, newcomers are frequently less interested in espousing a vegetarian identity than in learning about vegetarian food options in grocery stores and restaurants. As a result, leaders generally try to embrace all changes in a positive direction, no matter how small, in the hope that someone who gradually reduces his or her meat consumption today may become an ovo-lacto-vegetarian and perhaps then a vegan tomorrow.[6] Most vegetarian leaders avoid uncompromising messages—such as those that demand immediate and complete change and those that do not acknowledge gradual changes as positive—which they perceive as likely to repel people who are learning about vegetarianism for the first time. Associating with a vegetarian identity may repel those who are just becoming interested, especially if they encounter negative reactions—such as jokes about eating rabbit food—from family and friends. Others may fear that by referring to themselves as vegetarians, they may be identifying themselves unintentionally with liberal politics and countercultural activities.

Collective identity can, however, function as a movement resource when positive identification with the movement's public image attracts new members. For example, vegetarianism—and especially veganism—is an aspect of the straight-

edge (sXe) movement, a youth counterculture that emphasizes a "poison-free lifestyle,"[7] which emerged out of the punk
rock movement of the 1970s and 1980s. The sXers often
dress in punk attire, have multiple body piercings, and draw
large black "Xs" on the backs of their hands (because night-
clubs sometimes mark underage club goers with a black "X"
to indicate that they should not consume alcohol) to represent their youth. Primarily representing a lifestyle of hard-core
music and bodily purity, sXe is also associated with involvement in animal rights, environmental, and (occasionally) anti-
abortion activism. Although most teens who adopt veganism
are not sXers, this counterculture has contributed to veganism's popularity: Some teens may be drawn to veganism because it shows commitment to sXe; others may adopt veganism as a sign of being "in" or part of a group.

The "desirability" of the vegetarian image—in this case,
among teens—can be a double-edged sword for the movement, however, if people who appropriate the image reap the
benefits of movement activities without making any personal
contributions to its success. Thus, a popular collective identity
can contribute to the "free rider" problem of inactive members that most movements experience.[8] Certainly, the vegetarian movement shares this problem. And as vegetarianism
becomes more trendy, we can expect the free rider problem to
increase.

Many people who adopt vegetarianism will free-ride because they consider vegetarianism a personal lifestyle rather
than a collective movement—a diet rather than a philosophically grounded way of life. According to Linda Gilbert, president of HealthFocus, a market research firm, "Concern about
fat is the number-one factor driving the mainstreaming of
vegetarianism,"[9] and health reasons for vegetarianism are less
explicitly "ideological" than ethical reasons. People who become vegetarians for health reasons are less likely to adhere to
a strict definition of "vegetarian" in practice, and it may be

hard to inspire health-motivated vegetarians to commit to vegetarianism as the meat industry develops less-fatty meat products that consumers perceive as healthful and nutritious. As a result, the broad, inclusive, health-oriented message that can initially attract new vegetarians and semivegetarians may backfire as the meat industry produces and markets products that address their health concerns.

By promoting primarily the health benefits of vegetarianism, organizations risk attracting adherents motivated only by self-interest, those who are not concerned with furthering movement goals. As a result, local groups that lack sufficient committed members suffer from leader burnout, and national groups that lack sufficient paying members do not have adequate resources to confront and respond to meat industry claims. In order to develop more committed, active members, it is important to strengthen vegetarians' commitment to a collective identity that considers vegetarianism a public moral good rather than merely an individual practice. The problem is how to do so in a way that still conveys an inclusive approach that embraces all personal changes in the direction of vegetarianism.

Vegetarian organizations, then, face the dilemma of how to divide resources between public outreach and the cultivation of future leaders. This problem is, of course, not unique to the vegetarian movement.[10] Movement organizations often find that they need to deliver a milder version of their message to the public than to their members. Sometimes, as in case of the vegetarian movement, the two versions conflict: encouraging members to become vegetarians to the fullest extent is the very message that would scare away many potential newcomers. In addition, the convictions of strongly identified vegetarians may seem overwhelming to newcomers, who may also see these vegetarians as incapable of empathizing with people who are just thinking about eating a little less meat.

Efforts to Balance Collective Identity
with the Public Promotion of Vegetarianism

The ultimate goal for vegetarian groups is for people to identify as vegetarians or vegans and to contribute positively to
promoting a more vegetarian world. In fact, as we have noted,
acknowledging the effect of social interaction, leaders encourage vegetarians to become exemplars for others to emulate. At
the same time, however, leaders encourage advocates and activists to focus on the changes people *have* made rather than
on the changes they have *not* made. In order to be a strong
example, it is important to be consistent in both beliefs and
actions. Most vegetarians have experienced comments by
friends, family members, or acquaintances pointing out some
inconsistency in their lifestyle practice. Most commonly, people ask ovo-lacto-vegetarians, "If you're a vegetarian, why do
you wear leather shoes?"

As people move toward veganism and become more strin-
gent in their practices, they appear more consistent to others.
This consistency can help strengthen their commitment; as
they publicly portray the *meaning* of vegetarianism, they may
incorporate the vegetarian identity into their personal identities. In striving toward this moral consistency, however, some
vegans become preoccupied with the animal by-products in
the foods they eat and the products they use. In many cases,
sugar, beer, and wine are processed with animal by-products;
tires and photographic film contain animal by-products as
well. Because of the gelatin used on film, some vegans refuse
to go to the movies; others refuse to kill mosquitoes.

Vegans who become preoccupied with avoiding all animal
ingredients can seem overly zealous to others. As Ball writes,
"There often appears to be a contest among vegans for dis-
covering new connections to animal exploitation. . . . This attitude makes us appear fanatical and gives many people an ex-

cuse to ignore our message."[11] Thus, vegetarian advocates and activists must walk a fine line, balancing practicality and moral consistency. In the *Vegetarian Times* article "More Vegetarian Than Thou," author Jim Mason articulates this dilemma succinctly: "If you try to be pure, they say you're a fanatic, but if you're not pure, they say you're a hypocrite."[12] This leads to a number of questions: Where does one draw the line? How pure is "pure"? When does consistency require so much time and effort that it takes away from time spent in movement activities? Within the movement, vegetarians challenge one another's moral consistency as well. In one sense, this encourages vegetarians to examine their behaviors and beliefs. But at what point does this encouragement become divisive?

Vegetarian leaders refer to the moral arbiters of purity as the "vegan police" or the "V police." The V police scrutinize and criticize others for their lack of vegetarian consistency; sometimes they seem to engage in one-upmanship to see who can be the most morally consistent. Leaders view the V police as typically newcomers—those who have not grasped more effective ways to motivate people to change. I have witnessed several minor instances of V policing, but the most notable instance occurred at the 1995 International Vegan Festival during a presentation by an invited speaker, physician David Simon of Deepak Chopra's Center for Mind Body Medicine. Speaking on Aryurvedic healing, a form of East Indian natural medicine, Simon commented that it was spiritually and physically more healthful for a person to eat a chicken dinner prepared lovingly than to eat a vegetarian dinner prepared hatefully. This moved several audience members to hiss loudly. Later, when I asked a number of leaders and other participants about their reactions to the hissing, most of them expressed embarrassment for the group, and I could find no one who would admit to having hissed.

As this incident suggests, tensions can arise about the question of how to move vegetarians to motivate nonvegetarians without diminishing their enthusiasm for the quest to become consistent exemplars themselves. Although there is no simple solution, leaders encourage advocates to embody the positive personal traits of compassion and kindness. As vegan author Victoria Moran states, "For me, the essence of veganism is compassion . . . not just compassion for animals, but all the way around."[13] In his presentation at a national conference, one leader put it this way: "If you want to see a vegetarian world . . . be the nicest, kindest, friendliest person you can be."[14] As we have noted, the strategy of encouraging vegetarians to become positive role models can help them not only avoid overzealous behavior but also attract potential members through social networks.

The vegetarian collective identity can have both positive and negative consequences in promoting vegetarianism. Although groups want to promote an inclusive vegetarian message that the public will grasp and find beneficial (that is, a message based on health), the development of a vegetarian collective identity requires identification with the various motivations, especially those related to ethics. Because they have a mission beyond their own self-interest, ethical vegetarians (especially vegans) are the least likely to backslide and the most likely to become involved in vegetarian organizations. Leaders do not want to dissuade newcomers by promoting a collective identity that they cannot yet relate to; however, they need to promote a collective identity in order to develop leaders and volunteers with enough commitment to contribute time and monetary resources to the movement.

Adopting a collective identity helps build this commitment to advocacy and action, but when strongly committed advocates become overly zealous and judgmental, it can hinder the successful promotion of vegetarianism. Vegetarian leaders try to solve this problem by encouraging advocates to treat humans in the same manner that they would treat animals—with compassion and kindness. As Marcus writes in *Vegan: The New Ethics of Eating*, "Whatever one's reason for becoming vegan, it is at bottom *an act of compassion*, and compassion can become an act of deep transformation. If you are what you eat, switching your diet remarkably changes who you are."[15]

7 The Food Industry's Role in Promoting and Gaining Acceptance for Vegetarian Diets

There is a lot of volume [in a vegetarian meal], yet a claim is made for "lightness." Such a meal offers a suggestion that we might after all obey the paradoxical modern and consumerist injunction, "Eat, eat, eat—but stay thin, thin, thin."
—Margaret Visser, "The Sins of the Flesh"

Shopping for vegetarian foods today is much easier than it was twenty years ago. Veggie burgers, "not dogs," and tofu can be found in most grocery stores, even in remote areas. Most communities have at least one local health food store, and many support a food co-operative (or co-op), making it easy to find vegetarian foods, organic produce, and bulk goods such as grains and nuts. Large mainstream grocery chains, such as Wegmans and Safeway, have "natural foods" sections, and large natural foods grocery store chains such as Fresh Fields and Bread and Circus are expanding. Even on-line, at such websites as Villageorganics.com and nomeat. com, consumers can easily purchase a wide variety of vegetarian specialty food items.

At the same time, restaurants are also offering more vegetarian options. Although there has been a slow but steady growth in the number of strictly vegetarian restaurants, a more marked trend has been the increasing availability of vegetarian meals, including ethnic dishes, in conventional restaurants. Mainstream restaurants often promote these items as "heart healthy" or "low fat" rather than as "vegetarian." In 1992, as a result of the findings of a Gallup Poll conducted for the National Restaurant Association, the organization advised its members to offer more vegetarian meals.[1] Over the past several years, many restaurants, including even some fast-food restaurants, seem to have heeded this advice. In addition, most colleges and universities, as well as many elementary and high schools, now offer vegetarian meal options.

In recent years, the vegetarian food industry has flourished. Concern about fat intake; the desire to consume more natural, less-processed foods; and interest in the potential health benefits of soyfoods all contribute to this trend. However, most people (80 percent, according to one study) who consume such meat alternatives as tofu and veggie burgers are not vegetarians,[2] and neither are many people who order vegetarian meals in mainstream restaurants. The vast majority of people who consume these foods are concerned with their personal health rather than with ethical issues associated with meat consumption or with association with a vegetarian identity.

In one sense, the wider availability of vegetarian products and entrées has made vegetarianism seem more acceptable and easier to adopt. Vegetarians are now less frequently asked, "What *do* you eat?" and less likely to have difficulty finding meal options when dining out with their meat-eating friends and family members. This increased acceptance and availability, however, has not led to a dramatic increase in the percentage of the U.S. and Canadian population that adheres to a vegetarian diet. It seems that "vegetarian" has simply become one more option, like "Mexican" or "Thai," on the menu. Instead of identifying as vegetarians, many people "eat vegetarian"—on occasion, for health reasons or variety. For some people, eating a vegetarian meal one evening may make them feel more comfortable about eating a big juicy steak the next. Occasional vegetarian meals, in other words, may help relieve the guilt associated with eating "unhealthful" red meat.

The mainstreaming of vegetarian foods in grocery stores, restaurants, schools, and even hospital food service provides an *opportunity* for the vegetarian movement to promote the benefits of vegetarian diets. Vegetarian groups can use the easy availability of tasty, low-cost, satisfying vegetarian meals as a key selling point to attract new members. The wide variety of these foods has helped remove the sense of deprivation that many people have associated with vegetarianism. The commercialization of vegetarian foods, which suggests that the food industry has co-opted vegetarianism as a menu choice, can have both positive and negative consequences for the vegetarian movement. It presents a strong opportunity for the vegetarian movement to capitalize on a cultural environment in which vegetarian menu choices are acceptable. But it may also serve to further dilute the vegetarian collective identity.

Vegetarian Foods Go Mainstream

Manufacturing and selling such vegetarian-friendly foods as veggie burgers and veggie hot dogs is becoming an increasingly lucrative business. Between 1996 and 1997, for example, meatless burger and meatless hot dog sales rose almost 13 percent.[3] Perhaps surprisingly, many vegetarian products sell better in conventional supermarkets than in natural foods stores. For example, Gardenburger's mainstream supermarket business is worth four times that of its health food store sales.[4] These products are widely available: A survey of twelve major supermarket chains, representing eighteen hundred stores, found that all carry veggie burgers and tofu and 67 percent sell nondairy milk products, such as soy milk and rice milk.[5] Supermarkets bring vegetarian products to a wide range of consumers who otherwise would not be exposed to them. Mainstream supermarkets can "normalize" these products, making them appear more acceptable, especially when they are displayed and advertised next to their meat counterparts.

Among the most popular of all of the "meat alternatives" are veggie burgers. Harvest Burger (now manufactured by Green Giant), Boca Burger, and Gardenburger compete with a variety of smaller brands for the consumer market. According to a survey by the Soyfoods Association of America (SAA), when choosing a meat alternative, consumers rank taste as most important, followed by price and fat content; convenience is also important.[6] Because the perception that veggie burgers are healthful is not enough to attract consumers, therefore, veggie burger competitors seek to convince their audiences that their products taste "as good as meat."

Harvest Burger, Boca Burger, and Gardenburger all attempt to evoke in their advertisements the sense that their products give people the taste that meat does but in a more healthful way. For example, for several years, in an appeal presumably directed at an older, more educated audience concerned with its cholesterol level, Archer Daniels Midlands (which manufactured Harvest Burger before Green Giant) advertised its product on Sunday morning's "This Week with David Brinkley," proclaiming, "Want the flavor without the fat? Get all-vegetable Harvest Burger for Recipes." Boca Burger advertises in Sunday newspaper coupon supplements with a big picture of the juicy burger accompanied by the claim "You won't believe it's meatless." And in 1998, Gardenburger launched a $14 million television advertising campaign featuring advertisements during the television show "Seinfeld."[7] The success of veggie burgers, the most mainstream of the vegetarian products (or "meat analogs"), suggests that people are willing to accept meat alternatives when they are promoted as tasty, healthful, and convenient—and when they are portrayed as more similar to than different from meat.

Increasing acceptance and consumption of soy products has also contributed to the mainstreaming of vegetarian foods. In the late 1990s, consumption of soyfoods—which include such products as tofu, tempeh, soy milk, soy flour, soy nuts, and meat analogs—rose dramatically. According to estimates from Soyatech, a soy protein consulting company, annual soyfood sales increased from about $300 million in 1980 to more than $1 billion in 1997.[8] Soy has come a long way from its singular association with tofu, which was once voted "America's most hated food," beating out liver and brussels sprouts.[9] According to the Soyfoods Center, tofu consumption is "doubling every three to four years"; soy milk consumption has increased more than 700 percent since 1985.[10] Soyfood sales continue to escalate, driven in part by the FDA's decision to allow manufacturers to make health claims on soy-product labels. An October 26, 1999, American Soybean Association press release gave the example: "25 grams of soy protein a day, as part of a diet low in saturated fat and cholesterol, may reduce the risk of heart disease" and predicted that U.S. soy-protein consumption could double as a result of these new claims.

The FDA's sanctioning of soy was followed by the USDA's March 2000 decision to allow 100 percent of the federal School Lunch Program protein requirement to come from nonmeat sources.[11] Prior to this change, public schools could fulfill only 30 percent of the protein requirement with meat alternatives, and many schools combined soy protein with beef to cut fat content and effect a 20-percent cost reduction.[12] This new regulation will most likely mean a wider availability of vegetarian foods in public schools with more children being exposed to them. With cafeterias serving more than 35 million subsidized meals a day,[13] this new regulation is likely to mean a boost in sales of veggie burgers and other soy products.

As vegetarian groups and soyfood organizations applaud these policy changes, the meat and dairy industries criticize them and work to protect their own interests. In response to the new federal School Lunch Program protein guidelines, for example, a spokesperson from the NCBA stated, "We feel that the USDA has been quite irresponsible. . . . Soy isn't really beef. . . . It is placing at-risk children at risk for nutritional deficiency."[14] And the National Milk Producers Federation filed a complaint with the FDA against the soyfood industry, claiming that the name "soy milk" infringes on the proper use of the word "milk," which the federation sees as denoting an animal by-product. According to an industry spokesperson, "Soy-based beverages are attempting to directly compete with dairy products and are inappropriately taking advantage of the familiarity [that people have with the word 'milk']."[15] We can expect to see more such challenges from the meat and dairy industries with the increased mainstreaming of vegetarian foods.

Veggie burgers and other nonmeat items appeal to a wide variety of people, most of whom are not vegetarians. As one Cape Cod restaurant owner put it, "I'm surprised. . . . A lot of middle-aged people are ordering the veggie burger."[16] As legitimizing institutions such as government agencies deem these products acceptable and desirable, we are likely to see them become even more widely available. In addition, a new trend is emerging: Large food corporations are buying out smaller veggie-oriented firms. In the year 2000, for example, Kraft Foods bought Boca Burger.[17] This, too, will encourage the normalization of vegetarian foods.

Vegetarian Foods in Restaurants and Institutions

Vegetarian foods have also become increasingly available in restaurants and institutions. Whereas manufacturers have largely advanced the availability of vegetarian foods in supermarkets, consumers have been the moving force toward the presence of vegetarian foods in restaurants and institutions. The growing presence of these foods counters commonly held notions of vegetarian foods as insubstantial, ascetic, and boring.

Because dining out is a social experience through which people interact and display their status to others, restaurants can play a large part in legitimizing vegetarian foods as cuisine. The status of vegetables, which has historically been lower than that of meat, is changing, as a wide range of culinary venues (from haute cuisine to fast food) accept, and sometimes even exalt, vegetarian alternatives. What was once seen as a mere salad, for example, can become a colorful feast of vegetables, legumes, and herbs.

Using detailed examples and colorful photos of successful creations, food service industry magazines, such as *Restaurants and Institutions* and *Restaurant Business,* seek to educate their readers about how to best prepare and present vegetarian entrées. In *Restaurants and Institutions,* for example, Janice Matsumoto writes:

> A variety of plate preparations allows vegetables to shine and keeps customers interested in the food. At Canlis restaurant in Seattle, Executive Chef Greg Atkinson has three requirements for his meatless entrees: Every vegetable must be the freshest available in season; the plate must include at least three different cooking styles (grilling, deep-frying, baking, etc.); and the plate must use strong colors to give eye-appeal (brown mushrooms, red and yellow peppers, greens, deep-red beets).[18]

Variety and aesthetics (not ascetics) are key: As Toni Lydecker warns her *Restaurant Business* readers, "Restaurants doing the best job of boosting vegetarian sales know that a great dish stands on great taste, not philosophy. Brown rice and bland tofu doesn't cut it anymore."[19]

Approached as a culinary exploration, a vegetarian meal offers both novelty and security: Vegetables offer a wide variety of colors, textures, and tastes, and—unlike unusual meats (such as brains, squid, and eel)—unusual vegetables rarely evoke uncomfortable, ambiguous, or averse reactions.[20] Interestingly, according to a *Restaurants and Institutions* survey, "those who eat out frequently and . . . those who are the most 'adventuresome' diners are among the most interested in trying nonmeat entrees."[21] As cultural historian Margaret Visser suggests, vegetarianism can be viewed as a modern response to dealing with the endless choices engendered by a consumer society that discourages the appearance of overconsumption.[22] Therefore, "adventuresome" diners can display their status by eating an ample-but-light exotic vegetarian meal.

Fast-food chains also have expanded their vegetarian options, but because most emphasize simplicity and convenience, selections tend to be limited. Restaurants such as Chili's, Denny's, and TGI Friday's regularly offer vegetarian options, and Burger King and Subway have experimented with adding veggie burgers to their menus. "Little Caesar's Vegetarian Guide," a brochure produced by the pizza chain in 1995, proclaims, "Little Caesars is proud to acknowledge that it offers many menu items that are suitable for vegetarians, even for those with the strictest standards." In contrast with many pizzerias, Little Caesar's uses no animal by-products in its pizza crust and offers a cheeseless pizza option for vegans.

Fast-food restaurants can play an enormous part in normalizing vegetarian foods for the public. But because they assume that most people—associating fast-food giants with meat—would not think of ordering a veggie meal from a fast-food chain, they assume that vegetarian items would not be big-selling items in their establishments. A survey of fast-food users found that these consumers are relatively disinterested in healthful or nutritious food.[23] Even chains that have offered intentionally veggie-friendly fare have had difficulty getting the ingredients right: Wendy's Garden Veggie Pita contained gelatin (produced from animal by-products) and Taco Bell's Veggie Fajita Wrap contained sauce made with chicken extract.[24]

In schools, businesses, hospitals, and other institutions, food services tend to cater to the needs and demands of the people they serve. In many cases in these settings, even a small group that makes demands for vegetarian options can have an impact. Many colleges and universities began to include vegetarian items on their menus as a direct result of student demand, and today virtually all offer at least one (even if only a pasta and tomato sauce dish) vegetarian option. As Chef Michial C. Neal explains, for example, Lynchburg College added a veggie option to its menu in 1997 because "vegetarians are probably one of the more vocal groups that dine with us, and this new line satisfies their requests."[25] With the increasing number of vegans on college campuses, food service directors find that by serving vegan meals, they can satisfy a larger audience—both ovo-lacto-vegetarians and vegans.[26]

Because, to date, no large-scale survey of vegetarians has targeted college students specifically, we have no firm figures on how many follow vegetarian diets. However, David B. Wasser's October 6, 1995, PCRM press release, "Survey Shows Vegetarian Food Catching on Big with Young Women," states that as many as 15 percent of women between 18 and 24 choose a vegetarian option on a regular basis. Although it is likely that not all of these diners are vegetarians, having the options available may make them more receptive to, or even more insistent on, the presence of vegetarian foods in the future. In fact, food service directors claim that recent college graduates are already demanding more vegetarian options in their workplace environments.[27] If this trend continues, we can expect the availability of vegetarian foods to continue to increase.

The Food Industry's Impact on the Vegetarian Movement

Certainly, the food industry's interest in vegetarian foods has played a significant role in the public's perception of these foods as normal and acceptable. Although nonvegetarians (and even some vegetarians) may still balk at plain tofu, nonmeat products that look and taste like meat are increasingly seen as healthful alternatives. Consequently, some nonvegetarians are coming to accept meatlike veggie products as a convenient, tasty, and cost effective alternative, and other nonvegetarians are beginning to enjoy vegetarian foods as a colorful, textureful, flavorful novel cuisine. Aided by changing government regulations that favor nonmeat protein sources, the food industry has brought vegetarian foods to mainstream America.

Although future surveys may reflect the influence of the increased availability of vegetarian foods on the younger population in particular, current numbers do not show a significant increase in the percentage of North Americans who identify as vegetarians. Many people seem to consider vegetarian foods, instead, as menu alternatives that extend their range of culinary choices. In the United Kingdom, sociologists Alan Beardsworth and Teresa Keil see this phenomenon as turning philosophically driven vegetarianism into the mere practice of vegetable-centered eating, with no identity component at all:

> The food manufacturing/retailing industry may act as a stabilizer, consolidating and "sanitizing" eccentric foodways by commercializing and exploiting them. . . . Hence a diluted, less morally charged form of vegetarianism may be generated commercially. This, along with new products, improved availability and more information, lowers the threshold of entry into vegetarianism (and even veganism) and hence mass recruitment can begin into a popularized set of foodways.[28]

The authors conclude that the commercialization of vegetarianism may lead to a weakening of vegetarian societies in the United Kingdom.

Now that by lobbying stores and restaurants to make more options available, vegetarian organizations in the United States and Canada have contributed to the presence and acceptance of vegetarian food options, these organizations are in a position to reevaluate their role in promoting the availability of vegetarian foods. Increased public acceptance of vegetarian foods offers a new set of cultural resources from which the vegetarian movement can draw to promote its message.

8 What Is the Future of the Vegetarian Movement?

The attitude towards vegetarianism in the last twenty years has certainly changed. In the 1970s and early 1980s when we did outreach booths, often people would ask us, "Why be a vegetarian?" We almost never hear that question now. Instead people come by and say, "I wish I could do that."
—Charles Stahler, "How Many Vegetarians Are There?"

In the late 1960s and 1970s—spurred by the hippie counterculture, by such seminal works as Lappé's *Diet for a Small Planet* and Singer's *Animal Liberation,* and by dietitians' and physicians' increasing acceptance of vegetarianism —the North American vegetarian movement gained significant momentum. Since that time—at least in terms of the percentage of the population that practices vegetarianism and that participates in vegetarian organizations—the vegetarian movement has changed little.

By holding conferences and distributing vegetarian information, vegetarian organizations such as AVS and NAVS tried to capitalize on the increasing public interest in and attention toward vegetarianism in the 1970s. In addition, both organizations helped to start dozens of local groups and began to produce their own publications. In 1975, NAVS sponsored the World Vegetarian Congress in Orono, Maine—the first international vegetarian conference held in the United States. A *New York Times* article about the event, complete with photographs and interviews with participants, reported that fifteen hundred people from around the world were in attendance. Summarizing the pervasive attitude of conference participants, the article stated, "Although they may argue over which brand of vegetarianism is the best, no one here seems to argue over one thing: their belief that vegetarianism is a mushrooming movement. They attribute much of this growth to young people, many of whom come to vegetarianism through yoga."[1] Although the 1970s was a decade of great opportunity for the promotion of vegetarianism, national organizations—which were just beginning to mobilize their resources—lacked the means to reach the many people who had both the interested and the will to change. Even today, the vegetarian movement lacks the necessary resources to spread its message and confront the meat and dairy industries directly.[2]

Perhaps the vegetarian movement missed a cultural opportunity to influence people's eating habits and consciousness more pervasively. But even if it had not, the movement would have faced a number of obstacles—created by its operating resources, strategies, and cultural environment—that have kept it from expanding.

Why Hasn't the Vegetarian Movement Had More Success?

The vegetarian movement has promoted vegetarianism by drawing attention to health benefits that have been confirmed by conventional scientific research. At the same time, thanks to more than two decades of movement lobbying, health food stores, restaurants, and even fast-food chains and conventional grocery stores continue to offer an increasing number of vegetarian options to the general public. If, then, it has become easier to follow a vegetarian diet, and mainstream science accepts vegetarianism as healthful, why aren't more people becoming vegetarians? I suggest two intertwined reasons: The vegetarian movement has proven to the public neither (1) that meat eating is imminently *dangerous* nor (2) that meat eating is *immoral*.

Endangerment Claims and Morality Claims

Although many people agree that consuming large quantities of meat can be detrimental to their health, far fewer accept that consuming small quantities can be harmful. Consequently, it is difficult to convince them that it is more healthful to eliminate than to merely reduce their meat consumption. In other words, it is difficult to convince people that the consumption of even a small quantity of meat is a *danger* to their, and especially their children's, health. In general, claims about society's problems tend to be particularly effective when they posit "intolerable risks to one's health or safety."[3] Claims that not only consumers but also nonconsuming bystanders are endangered can be even more successful. For example, the resurgence of the controversy over cigarette smoking emerged in the 1980s when scientific evidence indicated that secondhand smoke was harmful to people's health;[4] the idea that children might be harmed proved particularly troubling.

Vegetarian leaders in North America have certainly tried to promote meat eating as a significant health risk. Lyman, for example, has crossed the country giving presentations on the imminent health risks posed by mad cow disease. At the 1995 International Vegan Festival, a year and a half before Lyman debated representatives from the NCBA and the USDA on "The Oprah Winfrey Show," he told his audience: "If you're going to have change, you've got to have crisis."[5] Mad cow disease, he predicted, would be the crisis that would move people to vegetarianism.

Public concern about the beef supply after the "Oprah" episode was short-lived: U.S. beef consumption did not fall in

1996. In contrast, however, as a result of major public concern about and government intervention in the spread of mad cow disease in the United Kingdom in spring 2001, according to one survey, the number of U.K. vegetarians increased from 5.4 to 12 percent.[6] Although it seems likely that some of these converts will prove to be only temporary vegetarians, the increase suggests that claims about the dangers of meat eating—especially if they are clear and present dangers that are supported by government and scientific authorities—can move some people toward vegetarianism.

The North American vegetarian movement has also had little success convincing people of the *immorality* of meat eating. Although animal rights sympathizers may be ripe for conversion, most people do not think of meat production as morally wrong. Unlike the foci of other social movement prohibitions—including smoking cigarettes, drinking alcohol, gambling, and engaging in adolescent sexual relations—eating meat is not socially regarded as a vice. Most people see eating meat—like drinking coffee—as an innocuous, "moral" pleasure. Moreover, in some groups, meat eating is an important signifier of social status: For people in lower socioeconomic classes, it can signify upward mobility, and for men, it can symbolize strength and vigor.[7]

People's desires for attaining pleasure and for enhancing their social status are likely to outweigh their moral ambivalence about eating meat. Interestingly, however, not all social groups perceive (or have perceived) vegetarianism as antithetical to pleasure and detrimental to their display of social position. In the hippie counterculture, many people practiced vegetarianism in the context of a form of hedonism that elevated the pursuit of pleasure to a moral good.[8] And among higher-income women, following low-fat, vegetable-centered diets is often requisite to achieving a desired signifier of their higher social class: thinness. Still, although some social groups perceive vegetarianism as pleasurable and consistent with high social status, most people seem to regard it as a feminine asceticism. Vegetarians are characterized by what they *don't* do, and for most people, this suggests control and restraint.[9]

Promoting Health Reasons and Moral Reasons

Generally, movement leaders perceive that some of the people who regard meat as a "moral pleasure" may be willing to give it up if they anticipate a direct health benefit.[10] The most common vegetarian movement strategy involves a slow educational process, centered first on health and gradually moving toward more overtly ideological concerns about the environment and animal rights. Unfortunately the movement's use of exemplary strategies that encourage people to change for their own benefit and that promote vegetarianism as a gradual path of self-enhancement do not seem to help build effective leaders and movement advocates; people who become vegetarians solely for self-benefit are not likely to contribute to the achievement of movement goals that benefit other humans and animals. Strategies that downplay the importance of identifying as a vegetarian in order to focus on the promotion of more vegetarian or plant-based diets may reach a wider audience, but they decrease the likelihood that vegetarian organizations will attract committed advocates.

Occasionally, however, in an effort to move people to consider their ambiguous feelings about meat eating, vegetarian organizations take the risk of promoting meat eating as an ethical issue. For example, several local groups took advantage of the popularity of the movie *Babe* by distributing information about slaughterhouses to *Babe* moviegoers. Some national organizations, particularly FARM, Farm Sanctuary, and Vegan Outreach, also encourage people to consider the relationships between human and nonhuman animals. Instead of creating advocates of the *abolition* of farm animal production, however, these efforts may create advocates of *reform* of brutal, inhumane slaughterhouse practices.[11]

Implications for Other Social Movements

Increasingly, *social* movements are concerned with changing *cultural* ideas, values, and attitudes. Cultural movements that require behavioral and attitudinal changes may find it difficult to convince potential members that they will benefit from these changes. For example, how do environmental organizations motivate people to feel that their daily actions can provide personal as well as collective benefits?

Moreover, moving people to make personal changes and recruiting people to contribute time and money to movement organizations are separate efforts that may involve conflicting strategies. Unlike coalition strategies that use preexisting infrastructures, such as membership in related organizations, cultural movements that cannot rely on social status identifications for recruitment are likely to rely on conversion strategies that use preexisting friendship and other social networks to attract new members. These conversion strategies are time-consuming, resource intensive, and potentially growth limiting. Instead of converting large numbers of people into faithful members, cultural movements may end up promoting *lifestyles* in which people use their purchasing power to demonstrate their concern for a particular issue (for example, by buying recycled paper napkins instead of regular paper or by buying hemp clothing rather than leather apparel). A person may use consumerism to express his or her self-concept or to reduce anxiety produced by a proliferation of choices in a commercialized society. A consuming lifestyle can become completely detached from any movement ideology; if a specific group upholds a certain lifestyle as desirable or if it comes to signify power and social status among a particular age group, it can become completely divorced from any ideological motivation.[12]

This consumeristic approach to movement involvement is not likely to bring about wide-sweeping cultural and social changes directly; however, it may contribute to the evolution of a cultural environment in which people support movement values without explicitly identifying themselves as members. Increased broad-based cultural support (even if it is only vaguely expressed as a willingness to buy vegetarian foods or recycled paper products) can afford movements more economic leverage when they make more specific demands for structural and cultural change. And, importantly, increased acceptance of basic movement ideas and the availability of related movement products can encourage people to see other movement claims as more valid and appealing. The increased availability and successful marketing of cruelty-free cosmetics (those that have not been tested on animals and include no animal by-products), for example, can create an environment in which consumers become more receptive to other animal rights movement concerns. Consequently, promoting diffuse cultural changes and lifestyles that are seemingly devoid of explicit movement ideology can help draw future committed movement constituents.

Still, there remains the possibility that promoting tenuous changes can sap movement resources that might better be directed toward effecting concrete ones. In the vegetarian movement, for example, because neither the strategy for converting individual vegetarians nor the strategy for effecting broad cultural change directly draws constituents who are willing to commit time and resources to movement activities, the combination of strategies seems especially draining. Lifestyle vegetarians who are motivated by self-interest do not tend to contribute time and money to projects that are intended to benefit the collective good. Compared with the animal rights and environmental movements, therefore, the vegetarian movement has weak organizational resources at its command.

Considering the Success of the Vegetarian Movement

Today vegetarian diets are much more widely accepted than they were two decades ago. With health organizations promoting the benefits of diets that include more fruits and vegetables and with the current emphasis on the benefits of low-fat foods, many people are considering how they might change their eating habits without giving up convenience and taste. The vegetarian movement has contributed to this healthful eating discourse by providing recipes and supplying nutritional information to people who want to eat less meat. As a movement, however, vegetarianism has maintained a marginal presence for almost two centuries. Because people generally view diet as a personal choice rather than as an expression of commitment to a collective effort, recruiting and maintaining members has been difficult.

The vegetarian movement and other movements whose activities are based on everyday life face a troublesome question: How can success be measured and articulated? Some cultural successes (such as the increased availability of vegetarian entrées at restaurants) are apparent, but because these changes are difficult to measure, they are difficult to demonstrate as benefits to potential members.[13] Without a specific set of long-term grievances, a series of winnable battles, in other words, how can organizations convince their constituents that participation is worthwhile?

This question is very difficult for the vegetarian movement to answer. Because grievance implies conflict, which vegetarian organizations tend to minimize in favor of consensus and solidarity, few vegetarian organizations express specific grievances. Instead of grievances, they emphasize gradual positive change and the increasing cultural acceptance of vegetarianism. Because the vegetarian movement makes few specific demands for social and cultural change, organizational successes are difficult to prove.

The first order of business for the vegetarian movement is to recruit new members. In order for the movement to mobilize for actions aimed at cultural and social change, its organizations must first persuade people to adopt both the philosophy and the practice of vegetarianism; movement participation requires a commitment to the vegetarian identity. Because "being a vegetarian" is a chosen rather than a status-based identity, a ready pool of people waiting to be mobilized based on this preexisting identity does not exist. By promoting vegetarian diets as a means of self-enhancement, as a personal path, rather than as an expression of commitment to helping other humans, animals, and the planet, movement organizations try to "plant vegetarian seeds" as widely as possible.

Without more vegetarians who are concerned with the ethics of the collective good (of both humans *and* animals) and are willing to participate actively in vegetarian organizations, however, what roles will vegetarian organizations play in the future? Currently, national organizations—emphasizing that social change occurs one person at a time—focus primarily on (1) producing educational materials for the general public and for local vegetarian groups and (2) conducting campaigns to increase the availability of vegetarian foods. Although the VivaVegie Society, FARM, Farm Sanctuary, and other groups also focus on promoting legislative changes, and VRG works to promote institutional changes, limited resources restrict the actions that can be taken. Increased links with the health food, animal rights, and environmental movements may well strengthen the vegetarian movement's influence and increase its resources in the future.

The future of the vegetarian movement seems to hinge on the ability to convince people that their personal choices can have a social impact and that this impact is worth not only their concern but also their individual sacrifice. Because food is central to people's lives—their memories, identities, and social relationships—changing both how they think about food and what they actually consume is a monumental challenge. The beliefs and strategies of the leaders of the vegetarian movement will play a significant role in determining whether vegetarianism remains a marginal, idiosyncratic, often temporary habit or a deeply embedded, socially acceptable, moral choice.

Appendix A

Methodology

This book relies heavily on movement writings and popular culture sources published since 1970; organization websites (see Appendix B) that address current vegetarian news and issues; and interviews with movement leaders and people associated with the promotion of vegetarian products, a survey of local vegetarian groups, and fieldwork at vegetarian conferences.

I interviewed thirty national and local vegetarian movement leaders, as well as other recognized activists. I also interviewed two people who are associated with businesses that promote vegetarian products and two people who are active volunteers in a national group.

I used a combination of target and snowball sampling to reach potential participants. I succeeded in interviewing at least one leader (for example, a president, executive director, or board member) in all but one of the nine national organizations; for information about Vegan Action, I relied on written materials provided by the group and my own field notes from a presentation given by the group's founder. I also interviewed leaders that I met at conferences and activists who were referred to me by other interviewees. My interviews, though essentially unstructured, included questions about the organization's activities and about the interviewee's activist history, involvement in vegetarian organizations, and views on the movement's current status (problems, goals, and future prospects).

Although this book's primary focus is national vegetarian organizations, it was essential to address movement activity at the local level as well. I started this project working on the assumption that local- and national-level activities are interconnected. In painting a broad picture of movement activity, therefore, I saw the need to address how this relationship operates. Thus my survey of local U.S. and Canadian vegetarian groups was born.

I began by using a list of Canadian groups provided by the Toronto Vegetarian Association (TVA), a list of vegetarian groups provided by VUNA and surveyed by Akers in 1992, a list of activists provided by VRG, a list of NAVS affiliates published in *Vegetarian Voice*, a list of "points of information" published in AVS's *Ahimsa*, and a list of groups mentioned in

151

Vegetarian Times to compile a complete list of local vegetarian groups in the United States and Canada. The names of groups compiled from *Vegetarian Voice, Ahimsa, and Vegetarian Times* (a total of 256) appeared in these publications between January 1995 and January 1996. I received responses from 156 groups, 97 of which turned out to be active local vegetarian organizations (the remainder were either dormant groups or animal rights groups). Many of these organizations also forwarded me copies of their newsletters, which provided another rich source of data about the local groups.

Between July 1995 and August 1999, I engaged in fieldwork at several regional and national conferences, including the International Vegan Festival, Vegetarian Summerfest, the Natural Products Expo, the New England Vegetarian Summerfest, and Louisville's Taste of Health Festival. I also attended public lectures outside these conferences, given by Robbins, Lyman, and other vegetarian advocates. My experiences in these settings proved to be a valuable resource for understanding (1) leaders' portrayal of vegetarian ideology and their attempts to build leadership and commitment and (2) advocates' assumptions about how personal, cultural, and social changes occur.

Appendix B

Vegetarian Websites

Listed here are websites for many of the organizations mentioned in this book, as well as additional websites that may be of interest to the reader. All websites were verified to be accurate as of January 2002.

American Dietetic Association (ADA)	www.eatright.com
Dairy Education Board	www.notmilk.com
EarthSave International	www.earthsave.org
FARM	www.farmusa.org
Farm Sanctuary	www.farmsanctuary.org
Howard Lyman	www.madcowboy.com
International Vegetarian Union (IVU)	www.ivu.org
North American Vegetarian Society (NAVS)	www.navs-online.org
People for the Ethical Treatment of Animals (PETA)	www.peta-online.org
Physicians' Committee for Responsible Medicine (PCRM)	www.pcrm.org
Toronto Vegetarian Association (TVA)	www.veg.on.ca
Veg Source Interactive	www.vegsource.com
Vegan Action	www.vegan.org
Vegan Outreach	www.veganoutreach.org
Vegan.com	www.vegan.com
Vegetarian Legal Action Network (VLAN)	www.veggielawyers.org
Vegetarian Pages	www.veg.org/veg/
Vegetarian Resource Group (VRG)	www.vrg.org
Vegetarian Times	www.vegetariantimes.com
Viva! USA	www.vivausa.org
The VivaVegie Society	www.vivavegie.org

Notes

Preface

1. See Joseph G. Gambone, "Octagon City," *American History Illustrated* 10 (1975): 11–15; David P. Edgell, "Charles Lane at Fruitlands," *New England Quarterly* 33 (1960): 374–377; Richard Francis, "Circumstances and Salvation: The Ideology of the Fruitlands Utopia," *American Quarterly* 25 (1973): 202–234; James Whorton, *Crusaders for Fitness: The History of American Health Reformers* (Princeton, N.J.: Princeton University Press, 1982); Janet Barkas, *The Vegetable Passion* (New York: Charles Scribner's Sons, 1975); and Anne Murcott, ed., *The Sociology of Food and Eating* (Aldershot, England: Gower, 1983).

2. For studies by sociologists in the United States, see Paul Amato and Sonia Partridge, *The New Vegetarians: Promoting Health and Protecting Life* (New York: Plenum, 1989). For studies by sociologists in the United Kingdom, see Alan Beardsworth and Teresa Keil, "The Vegetarian Option: Varieties, Conversions, Motives, and Careers," *Sociological Review* 40 (1992): 253–293. For research by nutritional scientists and dietitians, see Johanna Dwyer et al., "The New Vegetarians: Who Are They?" *Journal of the American Dietetic Association* 62 (1973): 503–509; Johanna Dwyer et al., "The New Vegetarians: The Natural High?" *Journal of the American Dietetic Association* 65 (1974): 529–536; Jeanne H. Freeland-Graves, Sue Greninger, and Robert K. Young, "A Demographic and Social Profile of Age- and Sex-Matched Vegetarians and Nonvegetarians," *Journal of the American Dietetic Association* 86 (1986): 907–913; Jeanne H. Freeland-Graves et al., "Health Practices, Attitudes, and Beliefs of Vegetarians and Nonvegetarians," *Journal of the American Dietetic Association* 86 (1986): 913–918; and Laura Sims, "Food-Related Value-Orientations, Attitudes, and Beliefs of Vegetarians and Non-vegetarians," *Ecology of Food and Nutrition* 7 (1977): 23–35.

3. Donna Maurer, "Becoming a Vegetarian: Learning a Food Practice and Philosophy" (master's thesis, East Tennessee State University, 1989); Frances Moore Lappé, *Diet for a Small Planet* (New York: Ballentine, 1971); Peter Singer, *Animal Liberation: A New Ethic for Our Treatment of Animals* (New York: Avon, 1975).

155

4. Ralph Turner and Lewis Killian, *Collective Behavior* (Englewood Cliffs, N.J.: Prentice-Hall, 1987), p. 223.

5. Judy Krizmanic, "Here's Who We Are," *Vegetarian Times* (October 1992): 72–80.

6. Linda Gilbert, "Marketing Soyfoods in the Next Millennium," *Third Annual Soyfoods Symposium Proceedings* (1998): 26–28.

Chapter 1: What Is Vegetarianism? And Who Are the Vegetarians?

Epigraph: Keith Akers, "Out of Synch?" *Pittsburgh Vegetarian Society* (newsletter) 3, no. 6 (1995): 1.

1. Ben Senauer, "Economics and Nutrition," in *What Is America Eating?* ed. Food and Nutrition Board, pp. 46–57 (Washington, D.C.: National Academy Press, 1986); Ben Senauer, Elaine Asp, and Jean Kinsey, *Food Trends and the Changing Consumer* (St. Paul, Minn.: Eagan Press, 1991).

2. Kurt Back and Margaret Glasgow, "Social Networks and Psychological Conditions in Dietary Preferences: Gourmets and Vegetarians," *Basic and Applied Social Psychology* 2 (1981): 1–9.

3. Thomas Dietz et al., "Values and Vegetarianism: An Exploratory Analysis," *Rural Sociology* 60, no. 3 (1995): 533–542.

4. Elizabeth A. Sloan, "Top Ten Trends to Watch and Work On," *Food Technology* 32, no. 7 (1994): 89–100; Janine Lopiano-Misdom and Joanne De Luca, *Street Trends: How Today's Alternative Youth Cultures Are Creating Tomorrow's Mainstream Markets* (New York: HarperCollins, 1997); National Restaurant Association, *Interest in Eating Vegetarian Foods at Restaurants: A Gallup Poll* (Washington, D.C.: National Restaurant Association, 1991).

5. American Dietetic Association (ADA), "Position of the American Dietetic Association: Vegetarian Diets," *Journal of the American Dietetic Association* 97, no. 11 (1997): 1317–1321; U.S. Department of Agriculture (USDA) and U.S. Department of Health and Human Services, *Nutrition and Your Health: Dietary Guidelines for Americans* (Washington, D.C.: USDA, 1996); National Institute of Nutrition (Canada), "Risks and Benefits of Vegetarian Diets," *Nutrition Today* 25 (March–April 1990): 27–29; Dietitians of Canada, "Celebrating the Pleasure of Vegetarian Eating" (available on-line at www.dietitians.ca/english/frames.html).

6. The grounds for vegetarianism may be much more complex than indicated by the motivations that most vegetarians articulate. For example, philosopher Michael Allen Fox (*Deep Vegetarianism* [Philadelphia: Temple

University Press, 1999]) lists ten arguments for vegetarianism. Interestingly, though, he does not include disgust at the thought of eating meat as a philosophical ground for vegetarianism.

7. Jennifer Jabs, Carol M. Devine, and Jeffery Sobal, "Model of the Process of Adopting Vegetarian Diets: Health Vegetarians and Ethical Vegetarians," *Journal of Nutrition Education* 30 (1998): 196–202; Rachel MacNair, "The Psychology of Becoming a Vegetarian," *Vegetarian Nutrition* 2 (1998): 96–102; Paul Rozin, Maureen Markwith, and Caryn Stoess, "Moralization and Becoming a Vegetarian: The Transformation of Preferences into Values and the Recruitment of Disgust," *Psychological Science* 8, no. 2 (1997): 67–73.

8. Vicki J. Hurlburt and Marilyn Nouri, "On Becoming and Being a Vegetarian: Decisions and Commitments" (paper presented at the Eastern Sociological Society meetings, Philadelphia, March 1998); Esther H. Kim et al., "Two Small Surveys, Twenty-five Years Apart, Investigating Motivations of Dietary Choice in Two Groups of Vegetarians in the Boston Area," *Journal of the American Dietetic Association* 99, no. 5 (1999): 598–601; Donna Maurer, "Becoming a Vegetarian: Learning a Food Practice and Philosophy" (master's thesis, East Tennessee State University, 1989); Randall F. White, Jennifer Seymour, and Erica Frank, "Vegetarianism among US Women Physicians," *Journal of the American Dietetic Association* 99, no. 5 (1999): 595–598; Judy Krizmanic, "Here's Who We Are," *Vegetarian Times* (October 1992): 72–80.

9. Krizmanic, "Here's Who We Are"; Chip Walker, "Meet the New Vegetarian," *American Demographics* (January 1995): 9–10.

10. Paul Amato and Sonia Partridge, *The New Vegetarians: Promoting Health and Protecting Life* (New York: Plenum, 1989); Maurer, "Becoming a Vegetarian."

11. Quoted in Maurer, "Becoming a Vegetarian," p. 81.

12. John Robbins, *Diet for a New America* (Waltham, Mass.: Stillpoint, 1987).

13. Francis Janes, interview by the author, San Diego, August 1995.

14. Stacey Vicari, interview by the author, Johnstown, Pa., July 1995.

15. Alan Beardsworth and Teresa Keil, "The Vegetarian Option: Varieties, Conversions, Motives, and Careers," *Sociological Review* 40 (1992): 253–293; Jennifer Jabs, Carol M. Devine, and Jeffery Sobal, "Maintaining Vegetarian Diets: Personal Factors, Social Networks and Environmental Resources," *Canadian Journal of Dietetic Practice and Research* 59, no. 4 (1998): 183–189.

16. N. J. Richardson, R. Shepherd, and N. Elliman, "Meat Consumption, Definition of Meat and Trust in Information Sources in the UK Pop-

ulation and the Members of the Vegetarian Society," *Ecology of Food and Nutrition* 33 (1994): 1–13.

17. Beardsworth and Keil, "The Vegetarian Option"; Jabs, Devine, and Sobal, "Model of the Process of Adopting Vegetarian Diets"; MacNair, "The Psychology of Becoming a Vegetarian."

18. Amato and Partridge, *The New Vegetarians*; Maurer, "Becoming a Vegetarian."

19. Kimberly D. Powell, "Lifestyle as a Dimension of Social Movement Study: A Case Study of the Vegetarian Movement in the United States" (Ph.D. diss., Department of Speech Communications, University of Georgia, 1992), pp. 91–113.

20. Quoted in Maurer, "Becoming a Vegetarian," pp. 55–56.

21. Jabs, Devine, and Sobal, "Maintaining Vegetarian Diets."

22. Amato and Partridge, *The New Vegetarians*; Beardsworth and Keil, "The Vegetarian Option."

23. Frances Moore Lappé, *Diet for a Small Planet* (New York: Ballentine, 1971); Peter Singer, *Animal Liberation: A New Ethic for Our Treatment of Animals* (New York: Avon, 1975); Erik Marcus, *Vegan: The New Ethics of Eating* (Ithaca, N.Y.: McBooks Press, 1998).

24. Keith Akers, *A Vegetarian Sourcebook: The Nutrition, Ecology, and Ethics of a Natural Foods Diet* (Arlington, Va.: Vegetarian Press, 1983), p. 201.

25. Jennifer Jabs, Jeffery Sobal, and Carol M. Devine, "Managing Vegetarianism: Identities, Norms, and Interactions," *Ecology of Food and Nutrition* 39 (2000): 375–394.

26. Amato and Partridge, *The New Vegetarians;* Beardsworth and Keil, "The Vegetarian Option"; Senauer, "Economics and Nutrition"; Senauer, Asp, and Kinsey, *Food Trends and the Changing Consumer.*

27. Michele Lamont and Marcel Fournier, eds., *Cultivating Differences: Symbolic Boundaries and the Making of Inequality* (Chicago: University of Chicago Press, 1992).

28. Margaret Visser, "The Sins of the Flesh," *Granta* 52 (Winter 1995): 113–131, quotation on p. 129.

29. Kurt Back and Margaret Glasgow, "Social Networks and Psychological Conditions in Dietary Preferences," p. 9.

30. Charles Stahler, "How Many Vegetarians Are There?" *Vegetarian Journal* 12, no. 4 (1994): 6–9.

31. V. P. Steeleman, "Attitudes toward Food as Indicators of Subcultural Value Systems," *Home Economics Research Journal* 5, no. 1 (1976): 21–32; Tony L. Whitehead, "In Search of Soul Food and Meaning: Culture, Food, and Health," in *African Americans in the South: Issues of Race,*

Class, and Gender, ed. Hans A. Baer and Yvonne Jones, pp. 94–110 (Athens: University of Georgia Press, 1992).

32. Robert J. Wolff, "Who Eats for Health?" *American Journal of Clinical Nutrition* 26 (1973): 438–445, quotation on p. 441.

33. Michael Goldstein, *The Health Movement* (New York: Twayne, 1992); Deborah Lupton, "Food, Memory, and Meaning: The Symbolic and Social Nature of Food Events," *Sociological Review* 42 (1994): 665–685.

34. Amato and Partridge, *The New Vegetarians;* Mark Messina and Virginia Messina, *The Dietitian's Guide to Vegetarian Diets* (Gaithersburg, Md.: Aspen Publishers, 1996).

35. Ann A. Hertzler and R. B. Frary, "Dietary Status and Eating Out Practices of College Students," *Journal of the American Dietetic Association* 92 (1992): 867–869; Jeffery Sobal, Dennis Revicki, and Bruce R. DeForge, "Patterns of Interrelationships among Health-Promotion Behaviors," *American Journal of Preventive Medicine* 8, no. 6 (1992): 351–359; Mary Zey and William Alex McIntosh, "Predicting Intent to Consume Beef: Normative versus Attitudinal Influences," *Rural Sociology* 57 (1992): 250–265.

36. Anne Sharman et al., eds., *Diet and Domestic Life in Society* (Philadelphia: Temple University Press, 1991); Julia Twigg, "Vegetarianism and the Meanings of Meat," in *The Sociology of Food and Eating*, ed. Anne Murcott, pp. 18–30 (Aldershot, England: Gower, 1983).

37. Carol Adams, *The Sexual Politics of Meat: A Feminist-Vegetarian Critical Theory* (New York: Continuum, 1991), p. 32. See also Fox, *Deep Vegetarianism.*

38. Deborah Lupton, *Food, Self, and Society* (London: Sage, 1996); Twigg, "Vegetarianism and the Meanings of Meat."

39. Susan A. Basow and Diane Kobrynowicz, "What Is She Eating? The Effects of Meal Size on Impressions of a Female Eater," *Sex Roles* 28, nos. 5–6 (1993): 335–344; Sally Chaiken and Patricia Pliner, "Women, But Not Men, Are What They Eat: The Effect of Meal Size and Gender on Perceived Femininity and Masculinity," *Personality and Social Psychology Bulletin* 13, no. 2 (1987): 166–176.

40. Kim M. Mooney and Joanne DeTore, "Perceptions of Women Related to Food Choice," *Sex Roles* 31, nos. 7–8 (1994): 433–442.

41. Beardsworth and Keil, "The Vegetarian Option."

42. About Women, *Marketing Food to Women: How to Reach the Growing New Women's Food Products and Services Market* (Boston: New Women, 1997); Nicki Charles and Marion Kerr, *Women, Food and Families* (Manchester, England: Manchester University Press, 1988); Marjorie Devault,

Feeding the Family: The Social Organization of Caring as Gendered Work (Chicago, Ill.: Chicago University Press, 1991).

43. Diva Sanjur, *Social and Cultural Perspectives in Nutrition* (Englewood Cliffs, N.J.: Prentice-Hall, 1982); Charles and Kerr, *Women, Food, and Families;* Rhian Ellis, "The Way to a Man's Heart: Food in the Violent Home," in Murcott, *The Sociology of Food and Eating;* Messina and Messina, *The Dietitian's Guide to Vegetarian Diets.*

44. Amato and Partridge, *The New Vegetarians;* Carol Gilligan, *In a Different Voice: Psychological Theory and Women's Development* (Cambridge, Mass.: Harvard University Press, 1982), p. 69.

45. Gilligan, *In a Different Voice,* p. 100.

46. Charles W. Peek, Nancy J. Bell, and Charlotte C. Dunham, "Gender, Gender Ideology, and Animal Rights Advocacy," *Gender and Society* 10 (1996): 464–478; Donna Maurer, "Too Skinny or Vibrant and Healthy? Weight Management in the Vegetarian Movement," in *Weighty Issues: Fatness and Thinness as Social Problems,* ed. Jeffery Sobal and Donna Maurer, pp. 209–229 (Hawthorne, N.Y.: Aldine de Gruyter, 1999).

47. Jeanne H. Freeland-Graves, Sue Grenninger, and Robert K. Young, "A Demographic and Social Profile of Age- and Sex-Matched Vegetarians and Nonvegetarians," *Journal of the American Dietetic Association* 86 (1986): 907–913; Sims, "Food-Related Value-Orientations, Attitudes, and Beliefs of Vegetarians and Non-Vegetarians," *Ecology of Food and Nutrition* 7 (1977): 23–25; Hurlburt and Nouri, "On Becoming and Being a Vegetarian"; Maurer, "Becoming a Vegetarian."

48. Peter Berger, *The Sacred Canopy: Elements of a Sociological Theory of Religion* (New York: Doubleday, 1967); Britta Wheeler, "Food as Cultural Artifact: A Look at Ideological Aspects of Food Behaviors," *Thresholds* 6 (1992): 68–74.

49. Freeland-Graves et al., "A Demographic and Social Profile of Age- and Sex-Matched Vegetarians and Nonvegetarians"; White, Seymour, and Frank, "Vegetarianism among US Women Physicians"; Dietz et al., "Values and Vegetarianism."

50. Freeland-Graves et al., "Health Practices, Attitudes, and Beliefs of Vegetarians and Nonvegetarians"; White, Seymour, and Frank, "Vegetarianism among US Women Physicians."

51. Freeland-Graves et al., "Health Practices, Attitudes, and Beliefs of Vegetarians and Nonvegetarians"; Tom McDonald and John Webster, "Nutrition Information, the Key to Better Diet, Better Health," USDA Release No. 0209.98, 1998 (available on-line at www.usda.gov/news/releases/1998/05/0209).

52. USDA, *Agriculture Fact Book 98* (Washington, D.C.: USDA, 1998).

53. Harvey Levenstein, *Revolution at the Table: The Transformation of the American Diet* (New York: Oxford University Press, 1988).

54. Marvin Harris and Eric B. Ross, "How Beef Became King," *Psychology Today* 12 (October 1978): 88–92; USDA, *Agriculture Fact Book 98*.

55. Stahler, "How Many Vegetarians Are There?"; Vegetarian Resource Group (VRG), "How Many Vegetarians Are There?" *Vegetarian Journal* 16, no. 5 (1997): 21–22; Toronto Vegetarian Association, "Vegetarianism—On the Rise," 1995 fact sheet.

56. Krizmanic, "Here's Who We Are"; Dietz et al., "Values and Vegetarianism."

57. Judy Jones Putnam and Lawrence A. Duewer, "U.S. Per Capita Food Consumption: Record-High Meat and Sugars in 1994," *Food Review* 18, no. 2 (1995): 2–11; Joel Gurin, "Are You a Semi-vegetarian?" *American Health* (July–August 1985): 37–43; Andis Robeznieks, "How Many Are There?" *Vegetarian Times* (October 1986): 16–17; "Survey Shows Interest in Vegetarian Items," *Restaurants USA* 11, no. 8 (1991): 20–21; Krizmanic, "Here's Who We Are"; Dietz et al., "Values and Vegetarianism."

58. Krizmanic, "Here's Who We Are"; Dietz et al., "Values and Vegetarianism"; Stahler, "How Many Vegetarians Are There?"; VRG, "How Many Vegetarians Are There?" 2000 update (available on-line at www.vrg.org/journal/vj2000may/2000maypoll.htm); Leslie Kaufman et al., "Children of the Corn," *Newsweek*, August 28, 1995, pp. 60–62.

59. David B. Wasser, "Survey Shows Vegetarian Food Catching on Big with Young Women," Physicians' Committee for Responsible Medicine (PCRM) press release, October 6, 1995.

60. Sloan, "Top Ten Trends to Watch and Work On."

61. Quoted in Walker, "Meet the New Vegetarian," p. 9.

62. Lopiano-Misdom and De Luca, *Street Trends*.

63. Peggy Noonan, "'Hey, Mom! I'm Going Vegetarian!'" *First*, December 18, 1995, pp. 99–100.

64. Gurin, "Are You a Semi-vegetarian?"

65. An essay from Max Weber,'s *The Sociology of Religion* (trans. Ephraim Fischoff [Boston: Beacon Press, 1922], p. 55) provides the language and theoretical basis for this dichotomy. Weber described two kinds of religious prophets: the "ethical" prophet, who demands obedience to God as a moral duty, and the "exemplary" prophet, who appeals to the seeker's self-interest and offers his life as an example of religious salvation for others to follow. We can use the same concepts without the religious terms and applications to describe social movements.

66. White, Seymour, and Frank, "Vegetarianism among US Women Physicians," p. 597.

67. MacNair, "The Psychology of Becoming a Vegetarian."

68. Quoted in Walker, "Meet the New Vegetarian," p. 9.

69. Rozin, Markwith, and Stoess, "Moralization and Becoming a Vegetarian," p. 68.

Chapter 2: Vegetarian Diets and the Health Professions: Historical Perspectives and Contemporary Issues

Epigraphs: Darla Erhard, "The New Vegetarians: Part One—Vegetarianism and Its Medical Consequences," *Nutrition Today* 8, no. 6 (1973): 4–12; U.S. Department of Agriculture (USDA) and U.S. Department of Health and Human Services, *Nutrition and Your Health: Dietary Guidelines for Americans* (Washington, D.C.: USDA, 1995).

1. Esther H. Kim et al., "Two Small Surveys, Twenty-five Years Apart, Investigating Motivations of Dietary Choice in Two Groups of Vegetarians in the Boston Area," *Journal of the American Dietetic Association* 99, no. 5 (1999): 598–601. See also Judy Krizmanic, "Here's Who We Are," *Vegetarian Times* (October 1992): 72–80.

2. Alan Beardsworth and Teresa Keil, "The Vegetarian Option: Varieties, Conversions, Motives, and Careers," *Sociological Review* 40 (1992): 253–293.

3. "Political Notes," *Time*, 52, no. 10 (1943): 17.

4. Michel Foucault, *The Archaeology of Knowledge*, trans. A. M. Sheridan (New York: Barnes and Noble, 1970), pp. 50–51.

5. "Trendscope," *Food and Nutrition News* 70, no. 1 (1998): 1.

6. ADA, "Position of the American Dietetic Association: Vegetarian Diets," *Journal of the American Dietetic Association* 97, no. 11 (1997): 1317–1321; American Heart Association (AHA), "Dietary Guidelines for Healthy American Adults," *Circulation* 94 (1996): 1795–1800; American Cancer Society (ACS), "American Cancer Society Guidelines for Diet, Nutrition, and Cancer Prevention," 1997 guidelines (available on-line at www.cancer.org); ACS, "Choices for Good Health: Guidelines for Diet, Nutrition, and Cancer Prevention," 1998 brochure.

7. It is important to point out that there is no comprehensive written history of the North American vegetarian movement. The secondary literature focuses on major figures within the movement and their personal philosophies. See, for example, Janet Barkas, *The Vegetable Passion* (New York: Charles Scribner's Sons, 1975); Gerald Carson, *Cornflake Crusade* (New York: Rinehart, 1957); Stephen Nissenbaum, *Sex, Diet, and Debility in Jacksonian America: Sylvester Graham and Health Reform* (Westport,

Conn.: Greenwood Press, 1980); Hillel Schwartz, *Never Satisfied: A Cultural History of Diets, Fantasies, and Fat* (New York: Anchor, 1986); and James Whorton, *Crusaders for Fitness: The History of American Health Reformers* (Princeton, N.J.: Princeton University Press, 1982). Colin Spencer (*The Heretic's Feast: A History of Vegetarianism* [Hanover, N.H.: University Press of New England, 1995]) offers a more global historical and philosophical account, and Joanne Stepaniak (*The Vegan Sourcebook* [Los Angeles: Lowell House, 1998]) gives a good overview of the organizational development of the North American vegetarian movement since 1960. I found no work that describes the chronology of the North American movement as a whole or that addresses how the general public experienced the movement in the nineteenth century. I cannot fill this gap here—I leave that important project to the historians. I offer, instead, some highlights of the movement and its leading historical figures.

8. Craig Calhoun, "'New' Social Movements of the Early Nineteenth Century," *Social Science History* 17 (1993): 385–427.

9. Richard Harrison Shryock, *Medicine in America: Historical Essays* (Baltimore, Md.: Johns Hopkins University Press, 1966), pp. 16–20; Michael S. Goldstein, *The Health Movement: Promoting Fitness in America* (New York: Twayne, 1992), p. 6.

10. Siegfried Giedion, *Mechanization Takes Command: A Contribution to Anonymous History* (New York: Oxford University Press, 1948); Ernest Lee Tuveson, *The Imagination as a Means of Grace* (New York: Gordian Press, 1974).

11. Robert H. Abzug, *Cosmos Crumbling: American Reform and the Religious Imagination* (New York: Oxford University Press, 1994), p. 171.

12. See, for example, William Metcalfe, "Bible Testimony on Abstinence from the Flesh of Animals as Food," in *Out of the Clouds: Into the Light* (Philadelphia: J. B. Lippincott, 1872).

13. Jayme Sokolow, *Eros and Modernization: Sylvester Graham, Health Reform, and the Origins of Victorian Sexuality* (Cranbury, N.J.: Associated University Presses, 1983).

14. Richard Harrison Shryock, "Sylvester Graham and the Popular Health Movement, 1830–1870," *Mississippi Valley Historical Review* 18 (1931): 172–183.

15. Joseph Gusfield, "Nature's Body and the Metaphors of Food," in *Cultivating Differences: Symbolic Boundaries and the Making of Inequality*, ed. Michele Lamont and Marcel Fournier, pp. 75–103 (Chicago: University of Chicago Press, 1992), quotation on p. 89. See also Carson, *Cornflake Crusade*, p. 52.

16. Clara Endicott Sears, *Bronson Alcott's Fruitlands* (Philadelphia: Porcupine Press, 1915); Louis Salomon, "The Least-Remembered Alcott," *New England Quarterly* 34 (1961): 87–97.

17. William Alcott, *Vegetable Diet Defended* (London: Concordium Press, 1844), p. 10.

18. Quoted in Goldstein, *The Health Movement*, p. 26.

19. Abzug, *Cosmos Crumbling*, pp. 177–181; Shryock, "Sylvester Graham and the Popular Health Movement, 1830–1870," p. 178; Carson, *Cornflake Crusade*, p. 19.

20. Ellen G. White, *The Ministry of Healing* (Mountain View, Calif.: Pacific Press, 1905); Barkas, *The Vegetable Passion*.

21. Goldstein, *The Health Movement*, pp. 44–45.

22. Neil Barnard, Andrew Nicholson, and Jo Lil Howard, "The Medical Costs Attributable to Meat Consumption," *Preventive Medicine* 24 (1995): 646–655, especially p. 647; Pamela Goyan Kittler and Kathryn P. Sucher, *Food and Culture in America: A Nutrition Handbook*, 2d ed. (Belmont, Calif.: West/Wadsworth, 1998), p. 97.

23. See, for example, Harold A. Kahn et al., "Association between Reported Diet and All-Cause Mortality: Twenty-one Year Follow-up on 27,530 Adult Seventh-Day Adventists," *American Journal of Epidemiology* 119, no. 5 (1984): 775–787.

24. See, for example, Mervyn G. Hardinge and Frederick J. Stare, "Nutritional Studies of Vegetarians: 1. Nutritional, Physical, and Laboratory Studies," *Journal of Clinical Nutrition* 2, no. 2 (1954): 73–82; idem., "Nutritional Studies of Vegetarians: 2. Dietary and Serum Levels of Cholesterol," *Journal of Clinical Nutrition* 2, no. 2 (1954): 83–88; C. L. Melby, G. C. Hyner, and B. Zoog, "Blood Pressure in Vegetarians and Non-vegetarians: A Cross-Sectional Analysis," *Nutrition Research* 5 (1985): 1077–1082.

25. Eliot Freidson, *Professional Dominance* (Chicago: Atherton Press, 1970).

26. D. A. Roe, "History of Promotion of Cereal Diets," *Journal of Nutrition* 116 (1986): 1355–1363, quotation on p. 1361.

27. James Whorton, "'Tempest in a Fleshpot': The Formulation of a Physiological Rationale for Vegetarianism," *Journal of the History of Medicine and Allied Sciences* 32 (1977): 115–139, quotation on pp. 121–122.

28. Johanna T. Dwyer and Jean Mayer, "Vegetarianism in Drug Users," *The Lancet* 2 (1971): 1429–1430, quotation on p. 1430.

29. Darla Erhard, "The New Vegetarians: Part One—Vegetarianism and Its Medical Consequences," *Nutrition Today* 8, no. 6 (1973): 4–12;

idem., "The New Vegetarians: Part Two—The Zen Macrobiotic Movement and Other Cults Based on Vegetarianism," *Nutrition Today* 9, no. 1 (1974): 20–27; I. F. Roberts et al., "Malnutrition in Infants Receiving Cult Diets: A Form of Child Abuse," *British Medical Journal* 1 (1979): 296–298; E. N. Todhunter, "Food Habits, Faddism, and Nutrition," *World Review of Nutrition and Dietetics* 16 (1973): 286–317. See also Gary Varner, "In Defense of the Vegan Ideal: Rhetoric and Bias in the Nutrition Literature," *Journal of Agricultural and Environmental Ethics* 7, no. 1 (1994): 29–40, particularly pp. 35–37.

30. See, for example, American Academy of Pediatrics, "Nutritional Aspects of Vegetarianism, Health Foods, and Fad Diets," *Pediatrics* 59, no. 3 (1977): 460–464; E. C. Burke and D. M. Huse, "Multiple Nutritional Deficiencies in Children on Vegetarian Diets," *Mayo Clinic Proceedings* 54, no. 8 (1979): 549–550; E. Zmora, R. Gorodischer, and J. Bar-Zin, "Multiple Nutritional Deficiencies in Infants from a Strict Vegetarian Community," *American Journal of Diseases of Children* 133 (1979): 141–144; and Roberts et al., "Malnutrition in Infants Receiving Cult Diets."

31. Erhard, "The New Vegetarians: Part One," p. 10.

32. Ibid.

33. Erhard, "The New Vegetarians: Part Two," p. 21.

34. Erhard, "The New Vegetarians: Part One," p. 8.

35. Mark Messina and Virginia Messina, *The Dietitian's Guide to Vegetarian Diets* (Gaithersburg, Md.: Aspen Publishers, 1996).

36. Charles Attwood, "When Vegetarian Families Encounter the Law . . ." *New Century Nutrition* (July 1996): 6–7.

37. See, for example, R. Bakan et al., "Dietary Zinc Intake of Vegetarian and Nonvegetarian Patients with Anorexia Nervosa," *International Journal of Eating Disorders* 13 (1993): 229–233; and Anthony Worsley, and Grace Skrzypiec, "Teenage Vegetarianism: Beauty or the Beast?" *Nutrition Research* 17 (1997): 391–404.

38. M. A. O'Connor et al., "Vegetaranism in Anorexia? A Review of 116 Cases," *Medical Journal of Australia* 147 (1987): 540–542; Donna Maurer, "Too Skinny or Vibrant and Healthy? Weight Management in the Vegetarian Movement," in *Weighty Issues: Fatness and Thinness as Social Problems*, ed. Jeffery Sobal and Donna Maurer, pp. 209–229 (Hawthorne, N.Y.: Aldine de Gruyter, 1999).

39. ADA, "Position Paper on the Vegetarian Approach to Eating," *Journal of the American Dietetic Association* 77 (1980): 61–68; idem., "Position of the American Dietetic Association: Vegetarian Diets," *Journal of the American Dietetic Association* 88 (1988): 351–355; idem., "Position

of the American Dietetic Association: Vegetarian Diets," *Journal of the American Dietetic Association* 93 (1993): 1317–1319; idem., "Position of the American Dietetic Association: Vegetarian Diets," 1997, pp. 1317–1321.

40. ADA, "Position of the American Dietetic Association: Vegetarian Diets," 1997, p. 1317.

41. Ibid., p. 1320.

42. ADA, "Dietetic Practice Group #14: Vegetarian Nutrition," 1999 (available on-line at www.eatright.org/dpg/dpg14.html).

43. USDA, *Nutrition and Your Health*, p. 8.

44. Michael Zimmerman and Norman Kretchmer, "Isn't It Time to Teach Nutrition to Medical Students?" *American Journal of Clinical Nutrition* 58 (1993): 828–829; Barnard, Nicholson, and Howard, "The Medical Costs Attributable to Meat Consumption"; Jane Brody, "Health Toll of Meat Diet Is Billions, Study Says," *New York Times*, November 21, 1995.

45. Myron Winick, "Nutrition Education in Medical Schools," *American Journal of Clinical Nutrition* 58 (1993): 825–827, especially p. 826; Robert F. Kushner, "Barriers to Providing Nutrition Counseling by Physicians: A Survey of Primary Care Practitioners," *Preventive Medicine* 24 (1995): 546–552.

46. Raymond H. Murray and Arthur J. Rubel, "Physicians and Healers: Unwitting Partners in Health Care," *New England Journal of Medicine* 326 (1992): 61–64; Dean Ornish, *Stress, Diet, and Your Heart* (New York: Signet, 1984).

47. "Avoiding the Surgeon's Knife," *Nova*, show #1818, television broadcast, December 1, 1991 (transcript provided by Journal Graphics); Dean Ornish et al., "Can Lifestyle Changes Reverse Coronary Heart Disease?" *Lancet* 336 (1990): 129–133.

48. K. Gould et al., "Changes in Myocardial Perfusion Abnormalities by Positron Emission Tomography after Long-term, Intense Risk Factor Modification," *Journal of the American Medical Association* 274 (1995): 894–901; Dean Ornish et al., "Intensive Lifestyle Changes for Reversal of Coronary Heart Disease," *Journal of the American Medical Association* 280 (1998): 2001–2007.

49. Tim Friend, "Patient Calls Ornish Program 'Miraculous,'" *USA Today*, September 20, 1995, pp. 1A–2A.

50. "Avoiding the Surgeon's Knife," p. 8.

51. M. L. Apte and Judith Katona-Apte, "Diet and Social Movements in American Society: The Last Two Decades," in *Food in Change:*

Eating Habits from the Middle Ages to the Present Day, ed. Alexander Fenton and Eszter Kisban, pp. 26–33 (Edinburgh, Scotland: John Donald Publishers, 1986); Warren J. Belasco, *Appetite for Change: How the Counterculture Took on the Food Industry* (Ithaca, N.Y.: Cornell University Press, 1993).

52. Belasco, *Appetite for Change*, p. 58.

53. Lappé, *Diet for a Small Planet*, 53–54, emphasis in original.

54. National Research Council, "Vegetarian Diets," *Journal of the American Dietetic Association* 65 (1974): 121–122.

55. ADA, "Position Paper on Food and Nutrition Misinformation on Selected Topics," *Journal of the American Dietetic Association* 66 (1975): 277–280, quotation on p. 279.

56. ADA, "Position Paper on the Vegetarian Approach to Eating," p. 64.

57. Suzanne Havala, interview by the author, February 1996. See also V. R. Young and Peter Pellet, "Plant Proteins in Relation to Human Protein and Amino Acid Nutrition," *American Journal of Clinical Nutrition* 59 (1994): 1203S–1212S.

58. ADA, "Position of the American Dietetic Association: Vegetarian Diets," 1988, p. 351.

59. USDA, *Nutrition and Your Health*, p. 8.

60. ADA, "Eating Well—The Vegetarian Way," p. 3.

61. Dietitians of Canada, "Celebrating the Pleasure of Vegetarian Eating," 1995 fact sheet (available on-line at www.dietitians.ca/english/frames.html).

62. American Academy of Pediatrics, *Guide to Your Child's Nutrition* (New York: Villard, 1999), pp. 80–81.

63. Judy Jones Putnam and Lawrence A. Duewer, "U.S. Per Capita Food Consumption: Record-High Meat and Sugars in 1994," *Food Review* 18, no. 2 (1995): 2–11, quotation on p. 4. See also Joel Gurin, "Are You a Semi-vegetarian?" *American Health* (July–August 1985): 37–43.

64. Barry Sears, *The Zone* (New York: HarperCollins, 1995).

65. Deborah Lupton, *Food, the Body and the Self* (London: Sage, 1996), p. 27.

66. Elizabeth A. Sloan, "Top Ten Trends to Watch and Work On," *Food Technology* 32, no. 7 (1994): 89–100, quotation on p. 99.

67. Quoted in Frank Schultz, "Milk Not the Best Drink: Group," *Janesville Gazette*, October 3, 1998.

68. ADA, "Position of the American Dietetic Association: Vegetarian Diets," 1997; According to the ADA, vegans—who consume no dairy

products at all—do not need to worry about getting enough calcium as long as they eat some calcium rich foods daily; see ADA, "Eating Well—the Vegetarian Way."

69. USDA, *Nutrition and Your Health*, p. 10.

70. Quoted in J. M. Lawrence, "Don't Have a Cow, Man!—Nutritionists: Dairy Critics Spout Udder Nonsense," *Boston Herald*, July 6, 1998, p. 5.

71. ADA, "Position of the American Dietetic Association: Vegetarian Diets," 1997.

72. Benjamin Spock and S. J. Parker, *Dr. Spock's Baby and Child Care*, 7th ed. (New York: Pocket Books, 1998), p. 346.

73. Jane Brody, "Many Experts Question Spock's Diet for Children," *New York Times*, June 20, 1998, p. A1.

74. American Academy of Pediatrics, *Guide to Your Child's Nutrition*, p. 187.

75. Health Canada, "Canada's Food Guide to Healthy Eating: Focus on Preschoolers," 1999 guide (available on-line at www.hc-sc.gc.ca/hppb/nutrition/pube/preschoolers/howpres.htm); Michelle Simon, "Book Review of *Mad Cowboy: Plain Truth from the Cattle Rancher Who Won't Eat Meat* by Howard Lyman with Glen Merzer," June 1999 (available on-line at www.vegan.com).

76. Kathleen Meister, *Much Ado about Milk* (New York: American Council on Science and Health, 1994). Authors such as Frank Oski (*Don't Drink Your Milk* [Brushton, N.Y.: TEACH Services, 1992]) and Robert Cohen (*Milk: The Deadly Poison* [New York: Argus, 1998]) have also written books on the deleterious health effects of consuming dairy products. Cohen, founder and executive director of the Dairy Education Board (whose membership he estimates at twenty-five hundred), started lecturing at vegetarian conferences in 1999 (see www.notmilk.com). The Dairy Education Board has filed a complaint against the dairy industry regarding a milk mustache advertisement that features "Dawson's Creek" star Joshua Jackson in a scenario that, the board claims, promotes sexual relationships between adult females and underage males.

77. "The 'Milk Mustache' Ads Are All Wet," *Good Medicine* (Spring 1999): 8–9; "PCRM Takes the Dairy Industry to Task for New Bogus Claims" (available on-line at www.pcrm.org/news/FTC.html).

78. Quoted in Meister, *Much Ado about Milk*. Available on-line at the American Council on Science and Health website: www.acsh.org.

79. "Anti-Dairy Group Opens Campaign Attacking Benefits of Milk," 1999 CNN report (available on-line at www.cnn.com).

Chapter 3: Charting the Contemporary Vegetarian Movement in the Social Movement Field

Acknowledgment: I thank Pam Monroe of the Calgary Vegetarian Society for providing me with Calgary mayor Al Duerr's press release of his October 1, 1995, World Vegetarian Day proclamation, as well as copies of media reports of the event.

Epigraph: Vegetarian Union of North America, "Guide for Local Vegetarian Groups: How to Start, Maintain, and Expand Your Local Vegetarian Group," 1995 booklet.

1. Steven Buechler, "New Social Movement Theories," *Sociological Quarterly* 36 (1995): 441–464.

2. Mario Diani, "The Concept of a Social Movement," *Sociological Review* 40 (1992): 1–23.

3. Personal communications with organization leaders.

4. American Vegan Society (AVS), *Here's Harmlessness* (Malaga, N.J.: AVS, 1964); Jay Dinshah, *Out of the Jungle* (Malaga, N.J.: AVS, 1967).

5. *VUNA Views* (1996).

6. Information about this publication is available on-line at www.ivu.org/vuna/foodfair.

7. John Robbins, *Diet for a New America* (Waltham, Mass.: Stillpoint, 1987).

8. Stacey Vicari, interview by the author, Johnstown, Pa., July 1995.

9. *EarthSave Newsletter* 1995:15.

10. Quoted in Clifford Rothman, "Last Frontier of Animal Rights? The Farm," *Los Angeles Times,* July 6, 1995, pp. E1, E7.

11. Information about this legislation is available at www.nodowners.org.

12. Michelle Breyer, "Serving Vegans at Every Meal," *Food Service Director,* April 15, 1995, p. 52; Leor Jacobi, "A Winning Program for Vegan Dorm Food," *Bay Area Vegetarian* (1996, annual): 12–17.

13. Matt Ball, "On Being Vegan," *Vegan Outreach Newsletter* (Fall 1996).

14. The response rate for the survey was 49.24 percent. Akers, in collaboration with other members of the Vegetarian Union of North America (VUNA), conducted a survey of local vegetarian groups in the United States and Canada in 1992 and found results similar to those reported here; see Keith Akers, "Survey of Local Vegetarian Groups," *VUNA Views* 3, no. 4 (1992): 1–6.

15. Ibid.

16. Alan Beardsworth, "The Management of Food Ambivalence: Erosion and Reconstruction?" in *Eating Agendas: Food and Nutrition as Social Problems*, ed. Donna Maurer and Jeffery Sobal, pp. 117–142 (Hawthorne, N.Y.: Aldine de Gruyter, 1995); Nick Fiddes, *Meat: A Natural Symbol* (London: Routledge, 1991).

17. M. L. Apte and Judith Katona-Apte, "Diet and Social Movements in American Society: The Last Two Decades," in *Food in Change: Eating Habits from the Middle Ages to the Present Day*, ed. Alexander Fenton and Eszter Kisban. pp. 26–33 (Edinburgh, Scotland: John Donald Publishers, 1986); Warren J. Belasco, *Appetite for Change: How the Counterculture Took on the Food Industry* (Ithaca, N.Y.: Cornell University Press, 1993).

18. Norbert Elias, *The Civilizing Process* (New York: Urizen, 1978).

19. Lawrence Finsen and Susan Finsen, *The Animal Rights Movement in America: From Compassion to Respect* (New York: Twayne, 1994), p. 44.

20. James M. Jasper and Dorothy Nelkin, *The Animal Rights Crusade: The Growth of a Moral Protest* (New York: Free Press, 1992), p. 178.

21. Finsen and Finsen, *The Animal Rights Movement in America;* Gary L. Francione, *Rain without Thunder: The Ideology of the Animal Rights Movement* (Philadelphia: Temple University Press, 1996).

22. Scott Plous, "An Attitude Survey of Animal Rights Activists," *Psychological Science* 2 (1991): 194–196; Judy Krizmanic, "Here's Who We Are," *Vegetarian Times* (October 1992): 72–80.

23. Robert Sanders, "For Those Who Cannot Speak: Political Behavior in Defense of Animals," *Humanity and Society* 19, no. 3 (1995): 59–69.

24. James M. Jasper and Jane D. Poulsen, "Recruiting Strangers and Friends: Moral Shocks and Social Networks in Animal Rights and Anti-Nuclear Protests," *Social Problems* 42, no. 4 (1995): 493–512; Kimberly D. Powell, "Lifestyle as a Dimension of Social Movement Study: A Case Study of the Vegetarian Movement in the United States" (Ph.D. diss., Department of Speech Communications, University of Georgia, 1992).

25. Michael S. Goldstein, *The Health Movement: Promoting Fitness in America* (New York: Twayne, 1992), pp. 44–45, 56; William C. Whit, *Food and Society: A Sociological Approach* (Dix Hills, N.Y.: General Hall, 1995), pp. 13–16.

26. Belasco, *Appetite for Change*, p. 224.

27. Goldstein, *The Health Movement*, p. 62.

28. *Health Science* (1996): 5.

29. Randy F. Kandel and Gretel H. Pelto, "The Health Food Movement: Social Revitalization or Alternative Health Maintenance System?" in *Nutritional Anthropology: Contemporary Approaches to Diet and Culture*, ed. Norge W. Jerome, Randy F. Kandel, and Gretel H. Pelto, pp. 328–363

(Pleasantville, N.Y.: Redgrave, 1980); Matthew Schneirov and Jonathan David Geczik, "A Diagnosis for Our Times: Alternative Health's Submerged Networks and the Transformation of Identities," *Sociological Quarterly* 37 (1996): 627–644.

30. Kandel and Pelto, "The Health Food Movement," p. 338.

31. Schneirov and Geczik, "A Diagnosis for Our Times," p. 631; Whit, *Food and Society;* F. G. Crane, "Profiling the Health Food Store Shopper," *Journal of Food Products Marketing* 2 (1994): 53–59; Jill Dubisch, "You Are What You Eat: Religious Aspects of the Health Food Movement," in *The American Dimension: Cultural Myths and Social Realities,* 2d ed., ed. W. Arens and Susan Montague, pp. 115–130 (Sherman Oaks, Calif.: Alfred Publishing, 1982), especially p. 127.

32. Esther H. Kim et al., "Two Small Surveys, Twenty-five Years Apart, Investigating Motivations of Dietary Choice in Two Groups of Vegetarians in the Boston Area," *Journal of the American Dietetic Association* 99, no. 5 (1999): 598–601. See also Krizmanic, "Here's Who We Are."

33. Rik Scarce, *Eco-Warriors: Understanding the Radical Environmental Movement* (Chicago: Noble Press, 1990); Krizmanic, "Here's Who We Are."

34. William A. Gamson, "Political Discourse and Collective Action," *International Social Movement Research* 1 (1988): 219–244.

35. National Pork Producers Council, *Porkfolio of Lean Routines* (Des Moines, Iowa: National Pork Producers Council, 1997).

36. Wendy Marston, "Beef Makes a Comeback," *Health* (November–December 1996): 34–38.

37. Laura Shapiro, "A Food Lover's Guide to Fat," *Newsweek,* December 5, 1994, pp. 52–60.

38. These writings are available on-line at www.ncanet.org.

39. Jeremy Rifkin, *Beyond Beef* (New York: Dutton,1992); Kathleen Meister, *The Beef Controversy* (New York: American Council on Science and Health, 1993); William T. Jarvis, "Why I Am Not a Vegetarian." Available on-line at the American Council on Science and Health website: www.acsh.org.

40. Michelle Mittelstadt, "Ranchers Have Beef with Magazine," Associated Press wire report, February 28, 1997.

41. Alanna Mitchell, "Veggie Month Dies in a Stampede of Beef," *Globe and Mail,* October 6, 1995.

42. Alberta Cattle Commission website: www.cattle.ca.

43. Quoted in Chip Walker, "Meet the New Vegetarian," *American Demographics,* January 9–10, 1995.

44. Walker, "Meet the New Vegetarian."

45. Quoted in *Calgary Vegetarian Society Newsletter* (1996).

46. George Gunset, "Oprah Airs Beef Fears, Draws Ire: Merc Cattle Prices Sink; Industry Upset," *Chicago Tribune,* April 17, 1996, pp. C1, C2.

47. Ronald K. L. Collins and Jonathan Bloom, "Win or Lose, Dissing Food Can Be Costly," *National Law Journal,* March 21, 1999, p. A21.

48. Howard Lyman with Glen Merzer, *Mad Cowboy: Plain Truth from the Cattle Rancher Who Won't Eat Meat* (New York: Charles Scribner's Sons, 1998).

49. Collins and Bloom, "Win or Lose."

50. Christy Lemire, "Cattle Raisers Set Up Hotline," Associated Press report, April 7 1999 (available on-line at www.plant.uoguelph.ca/riskcomm/archives/animalnet/1999/4-1999/an-07-99-ol.txt).

51. Movement leaders tread lightly with respect to this subject, but several people have mentioned to me that personality and ideological conflicts have existed among movement leaders since the 1970s. At conferences, leaders from the various organizations are careful not to allow these differences to surface.

52. VRG offers its quarterly *Vegetarian Journal* as an incentive for membership; the journal provides current health and nutrition news and abstracts of research in nutrition journals that are much more scientific in tone than the health-related articles in the mass-marketed *Vegetarian Times.* NAVS has increasingly professionalized its publication (*Vegetarian Voice*) with well-researched articles on the health, environmental, and ethical aspects of vegetarianism, and VRG (one of the larger vegetarian groups) attracts many interested parties by offering its journal to members.

Chapter 4: Vegetarianism: Expressions of Ideology in Vegetarian Organizations

Epigraph: Stanley Sapon, "What's in a Name? Vegetarianism's Past, Present, and Future: A Linguistic and Behavioral Appraisal" (paper presented at Vegetarian Summerfest, Johnstown, Pa., August 2, 1996). Sapon's speech was excerpted in the New York City alternative publication *Satya* (November 1996): 16, and reprinted in full in *Vegetarian Voice* (January 1997): 12–17 and *European Vegetarian Union News* no. 3 (1996): Having struck a chord with vegetarian leaders and advocates who were grappling with how to apply the vegetarian ideology to their organizational activities, Sapon's paper sparked much Internet discussion and many letters to the editor.

1. Herbert Blumer, "Collective Behavior," in *Principles of Sociology*, ed. Alfred McClung Lee, pp. 210–211 (New York: Barnes and Noble, 1939).

2. Clifford Geertz, *The Interpretation of Cultures* (New York: Basic Books, 1964); Gary T. Marx and Douglas McAdam, *Collective Behavior and Social Movements: Process and Structure* (Englewood Cliffs, N.J.: Prentice-Hall, 1994), p. 31; Rhys H. Williams, "Movement Dynamics and Social Change: Transforming Fundamentalist Ideology and Organizations," in *Accounting for Fundamentalisms: The Dynamic Character of Movements*, ed. Martin E. Marty and R. Scott Appleby, pp. 725–828 (Chicago: University of Chicago Press, 1994).

3. I use a simplistic identification of these arguments as vegetarian organizations usually do. Philosophically and historically, the arguments can be considered with much more complexity, as Michael Allen Fox does in his ten arguments for vegetarianism in *Deep Vegetarianism* (Philadelphia: Temple University Press, 1999).

4. Albert Schweitzer, *The Philosophy of Civilization*, trans. C. T. Campion (New York: Macmillan, 1949).

5. Colin Spencer, *The Heretic's Feast: A History of Vegetarianism* (Hanover, N.H.: University Press of New England, 1995), pp. 33–68; Jon Gregerson, *Vegetarianism: A History* (Fremont, Calif.: Jain Publishing, 1994), pp. 5–12.

6. Tom Regan, *The Case for Animal Rights* (Berkeley: University of California Press, 1983).

7. Gary L. Francione, *Rain without Thunder: The Ideology of the Animal Rights Movement* (Philadelphia: Temple University Press, 1996), p. 16.

8. Peter Singer, *Animal Liberation: A New Ethic for Our Treatment of Animals* (New York: Avon, 1975); James M. Jasper and Dorothy Nelkin, *The Animal Rights Crusade: The Growth of a Moral Protest* (New York: Free Press, 1992), p. 90.

9. Singer, *Animal Liberation*, pp. 7, 167.

10. Carol Adams, *The Sexual Politics of Meat: A Feminist-Vegetarian Critical Theory* (New York: Continuum, 1991); Marjorie Spiegel, *The Dreaded Comparison: Human and Animal Slavery* (Philadelphia: New Society Publishers, 1988).

11. Adams, *The Sexual Politics of Meat*, pp. 34, 37.

12. Ibid., pp. 47–62.

13. Spiegel, *The Dreaded Comparison*, p. 24.

14. Julia Twigg, "Food for Thought: Purity and Vegetarianism," *Religion* 9 (1979): 13–35.

15. Richard Bargen, *The Vegetarian's Self-Defense Manual* (Wheaton, Ill.: Theosophical Publishing House, 1979), p. 4.

16. Spencer, *The Heretic's Feast,* pp. 33–68.

17. Barbara Parham, *What's Wrong with Eating Meat?* (Denver, Colo.: Ananda Marga Publications, 1979), p. 57.

18. Ibid., pp. 25–26.

19. Spencer, *The Heretic's Feast,* p. 50.

20. John Robbins, *Diet for a New America* (Waltham, Mass.: Stillpoint, 1987), p. 156.

21. Victoria Moran, *Compassion: The Ultimate Ethic* (Wellingborough, England: Thorsons, 1985), p. 68.

22. Rudolph Ballentine, *Transition to Vegetarianism: An Evolutionary Step* (Honesdale, Pa.: Himalayan Press, 1987), pp. 72–73.

23. Billy Ray Boyd, *For the Vegetarian in You* (San Francisco: Taterhill Press, 1987), p. 21.

24. Jim Mason and Peter Singer, *Animal Factories* (New York: Harmony Books, 1990), p. 188.

25. See Neil Barnard, Andrew Nicholson, and Jo Lil Howard, "The Medical Costs Attributable to Meat Consumption," *Preventive Medicine* 24 (1995): 646–655; *Farm Report,* "Farm Subsidies" issue (Winter 1996): 8.

26. Francis Moore Lappé, *Diet for a Small Planet* (New York: Ballentine, 1971) p. 8, emphasis in original.

27. Boyd, *For the Vegetarian in You,* p. 21, emphasis in original.

28. Keith Akers, *A Vegetarian Sourcebook: The Nutrition, Ecology, and Ethics of a Natural Foods Diet* (Arlington, Va: Vegetarian Press, 1983), p. 84.

29. Robbins, *Diet for a New America,* p. 35.

30. Field notes, John Robbins presentation, Louisville, March 27, 1996.

31. Animal bones are sometimes used in sugar processing.

32. Akers, *A Vegetarian Sourcebook,* p. 151.

33. Spencer, *A Heretic's Feast,* p. 317.

34. Keith Akers, interview by the author, San Diego, August 1996.

35. NAVS, "About NAVS," *Vegetarian Voice* 24, no. 3 (Fall 1999): 2.

36. "What Is VUNA?" *VUNA Views* 6, no. 2 (Spring 1996): 7.

37. Field notes, Vegetarian Summerfest, Johnstown, Pa., 1996.

38. Karl R. Kunkel, "Down on the Farm: Rationale Expansion in the Construction of Factory Farming as a Social Problem," in *Images of Issues: Typifying Contemporary Social Problems,* 2d ed., ed. Joel Best, pp. 239–255 (Hawthorne, N.Y.: Aldine de Gruyter, 1995).

39. Field notes, Vegetarian Summerfest, 1995.

40. Stanley Sapon, "What's in a Name? Vegetarianism's Past, Present, and Future: A Linguistic and Behavioral Appraisal" (paper presented at Vegetarian Summerfest, Johnstown, Pa., on August 2, 1996).

41. NAVS, *Vegetarian Voice* (1997): 17.
42. Sapon, "What's in a Name?"
43. Ibid.
44. Ibid.
45. Stanley Sapon, letter to the editor, *Vegetarian Voice* (1997).
46. Keith Akers, letter to the author, 1996.
47. Sapon, letter to the editor, 1997 (same as #45, above).

Chapter 5: The Beliefs and Strategies of Vegetarian Movement Leaders

Acknowledgment: I thank Liege Weill of VEGANAT for helping me find information on the Vegetarian Legal Awareness Network.

Epigraph: Field notes, Vegetarian Summerfest, 1996.

1. On material and human resources, see John D. McCarthy and Mayer Zald, "Resource Mobilization and Social Movements: A Partial Theory, " *American Journal of Sociology* 82 (1976): 1212–1241; on political constraints, see Gary T. Marx and Douglas McAdam, *Collective Behavior and Social Movements: Process and Structure* (Englewood Cliffs, N.J.: Prentice-Hall, 1994), pp. 108–109; and on group decision-making activities, see Gary L. Downey, "Ideology and the Clamshell Identity: Organizational Dilemmas in the Anti-Nuclear Power Movement," *Social Problems* 33 (1986): 357–373.

2. Keith Akers, *A Vegetarian Sourcebook: The Nutrition, Ecology, and Ethics of a Natural Foods Diet* (Arlington, Va.: Vegetarian Press, 1983), p. 206.

3. Howard Lyman, "Voice for a Viable Future," audiotape (Santa Cruz, Calif.: EarthSave Foundation, n.d.).

4. Field notes, Vegetarian Summerfest, 1995.

5. Esther H. Kim et al., "Two Small Surveys, Twenty-five Years Apart, Investigating Motivations of Dietary Choice in Two Groups of Vegetarians in the Boston Area," *Journal of the American Dietetic Association* 99 (1999): 598–601; Judy Krizmanic, "Here's Who We Are," *Vegetarian Times* (October 1992): 72–80.

6. Field notes, Vegetarian Summerfest, 1995.

7. Donna Maurer, "Too Skinny or Vibrant and Healthy? Weight Management in the Vegetarian Movement," in *Weighty Issues: Fatness and Thinness as Social Problems*, ed. Jeffery Sobal and Donna Maurer, pp. 209–229 (Hawthorne, N.Y.: Aldine de Gruyter, 1999).

8. Jennifer Brown, "Summerfest Points to Ponder," *The Grapevine* (newsletter of the Triangle Vegetarian Society) 9, no. 4 (1995): 11.

9. Field notes, Vegetarian Summerfest, 1995.

10. Peter McQueen (lecture delivered at the International Vegan Festival, San Diego, July 1995), AVS videotape.

11. Stacey Vicari (lecture delivered at the International Vegan Festival, San Diego, July 1995), AVS videotape.

12. Pamela Rice, telephone interview by the author, February 1996.

13. Field notes, Vegetarian Summerfest, 1995.

14. Matt Ball, telephone interview by the author, September 1996.

15. Stacey Vicari, interview by the author, Johnstown, Pa., July 1995.

16. Leor Jacobi, "A Winning Program for Vegan Dorm Food," *Bay Area Vegetarian* (1996, annual): 12–17.

17. Ball interview.

18. Susan Campbell and Todd Winant, *Healthy School Lunch Action Guide* (Santa Cruz, Calif.: EarthSave International, 1994), p. 58.

19. Rice interview.

20. Peter Singer, *Animal Liberation: A New Ethic for Our Treatment of Animals* (New York: Avon, 1975), pp. 181–182.

21. Judy Krizmanic, *A Teen's Guide to Going Vegetarian* (New York: Puffin Books, 1994), p. 66.

22. Field notes, Vegetarian Summerfest, 1995.

23. Dean Ornish, "Change Your Diet, Change Your Life," *Bay Area Vegetarian* (1995, annual): 36–41, quotation on page 38.

24. Karen Iacobbo and Michael Gibson, *Vegetarian Magic in Three Easy Steps: Change Your Mind, Change the Menu* (Providence, R.I.: American Lyceum Press, 1996), p. 15.

25. "How Meat Kills . . . and Why Many People Don't Eat It," *Vegetarian Connection* (newsletter of the Vegetarian Society of Central Florida) (March–April 1995): 7.

26. For an interesting article on this phenomenon from a psychological perspective, see Scott Plous, "Psychological Mechanisms in the Human Use of Animals," *Journal of Social Issues* 49 (1993): 11–52.

27. Iacobbo and Gibson, *Vegetarian Magic in Three Easy Steps,* p. 90.

28. Michael Klaper, *Vegan Nutrition: Pure and Simple,* 3d ed. (Maui, Hawaii: Gentle World, 1994), p. 21.

29. Marcella M. Modugno, "A Little Can Mean a Lot—the Truth about Vitamin B-12," *Viva Vine* 66, no. 1 (1997): 1, 12–13.

30. Keith Akers, interview by the author, San Diego, August 1995.

31. Klaper, *Vegan Nutrition,* p. 42.

32. For example, see Akers, *A Vegetarian Sourcebook;* Erik Marcus, *Vegan: The New Ethics of Eating* (Ithaca, N.Y.: McBooks Press, 1998); Frances Moore Lappé, *Diet for a Small Planet* (New York: Ballentine,

1971); and Sharon K. Yntema, *Vegetarian Children: A Supportive Guide for Parents* (Ithaca, N.Y.: McBooks Press, 1987). For an overview, see Donna Maurer, "Meat as a Social Problem: Rhetorical Strategies in the Contemporary Vegetarian Literature," in *Eating Agendas: Food and Nutrition as Social Problems*, ed. Donna Maurer and Jeffery Sobal, pp. 143–163 (Hawthorne, N.Y.: Aldine de Gruyter, 1995).

33. Richard Bargen, *The Vegetarian's Self-Defense Manual* (Wheaton, Ill.: Theosophical Publishing House, 1979), p. 31.

34. Jon Wynne-Tyson, *Food for a Future: The Ecological Priority of a Humane Diet* (London: Davis-Poynter, 1975).

35. *Viva Vine* (1996): 3.

36. Pamela Rice, "VivaVegie Plants Doubt in the Minds of San Gennero Feast-goers," *The VivaVine* 5, no. 3 (1996): 1, 3.

37. "Pork Power," *60 Minutes*, December 22, 1996, television broadcast (transcript provided by Burrelle's Information Services).

38. Quoted in Donald P. Baker, "N.C. Mega-Hog Farm Runs Afoul of Neighbors," *Washington Post*, December 22, 1996, p. B3.

39. Ball interview.

40. *Sanctuary News* (Summer 1995): 2.

41. A large archive of newspaper and magazine articles about the trial, as well as transcripts of court testimonies and interviews with those who testified, is available at www.mcspotlight.org.

42. Kyle Pope, "Turning the Tables: Charged with Libel, Pair of Activists Puts McDonald's on Grill," *Wall Street Journal*, July 18, 1995, pp. A1, A5.

43. Cres Vellucci, "How to Be an Activist: Reports from World Anti-McDonald's Day, October 16," *Satya* 3 (May 1996): 19.

44. Ibid.

45. Susan Skeels Sams, letter, *Vegetarian Society of Toledo Newsletter* 7, no. 6 (1995): 3.

46. Debra Wasserman, interview by the author, Baltimore, September 1995.

47. Suzanne Havala, "Update: USDA School Meals Initiative for Healthy Children," *Vegetarian Journal* 13 (November–December 1994): 7–9.

48. Suzanne Havala, interview by the author, February 1996.

49. Charles Patterson, "Economic Justice," *Viva Vine* 5, no. 2 (1996): 4–5.

50. "Veggie Bus Driver Wins Legal Battle," *VivaVine* 6, no. 1 (January–February 1997). Available on-line at vivavegie.org/vvi/vva/vvi24/news.html.

51. Quotation available on-line at www.veggielawyers.org.

52. Emphasis in original.

53. "Vegan Action Hires Executive Director," *Vegan News* (Fall 1998): 1.

54. Freya Dinshah, "The Value of Freedom," *Ahimsa* 37, no. 4 (1996): 20.

55. George Eisman with Matt Ball and Anne Green, *The Most Noble Diet: Food Selection and Ethics* (Burdett, N.Y.: Diet Ethics, 1994), p. 56.

Chapter 6: Organizational Strategy in Action: Promoting a Vegetarian Collective Identity

Epigraph: Matt Ball, Jack Norris, and Anne Green, "Tips for Spreading Veganism," 1999 Vegan Outreach brochure.

1. Charles Stahler, "How Many Vegetarians Are There?" *Vegetarian Journal* 12 (July–August 1994): 6–9.

2. Audrey Nickel, "The Times, They Are A-Changin' (Aren't They?)," *The Grapevine* (newsletter of the Triangle Vegetarian Society) 9 (April 1995): 1, 15.

3. Hank Johnston, Enrique Laraña, and Joseph Gusfield, "Identities, Grievances, and New Social Movements," in *New Social Movements: From Ideology to Identity*, ed. Enrique Laraña, Hank Johnston, and Joseph Gusfield, pp. 3–35 (Philadelphia: Temple University Press, 1994).

4. *Vegan News* (1995): 2.

5. Although most of the many people I met at conferences were on the path to vegetarianism, I came across a few less-than-enthusiastic meat-eating spouses.

6. Victoria Moran, *Compassion: The Ultimate Ethic* (Wellingborough, England: Thorsons, 1985), p. 44.

7. Elizabeth Shepard, "Walking a Straight Line," *React* (a supplement to *The Patriot-News*), December 2–8, 1996, pp. 8–9.

8. Debra Friedman and Doug McAdam, "Collective Identity and Activism: Networks, Choices, and the Life of a Social Movement" in *Frontiers in Social Movement Theory*, ed. Aldon D. Morris and Carol McClurg Mueller, pp. 156–173 (New Haven, Conn.: Yale University Press, 1992).

9. Quoted in Chip Walker, "Meet the New Vegetarian," *American Demographics* (January 1995): 9–10.

10. Timothy J. Kubal, "The Presentation of Political Self: Cultural Resonance and the Construction of Collective Action Frames," *Sociological Quarterly* 39 (1998): 539–554.

11. Matt Ball, "Activism and Veganism Reconsidered: Personal Thoughts at the New Millennium" (manuscript, n.d.).

12. Quoted in Max Friedman, "More Vegetarian Than Thou," *Vegetarian Times* (September 1995): 59–64, quotation on p. 62.
13. Quoted in ibid.
14. Field notes, 1995.
15. Erik Marcus, *Vegan: The New Ethics of Eating* (Ithaca, N.Y.: Mc-Books Press, 1998), p. 191.

Chapter 7: The Food Industry's Role in Promoting and Gaining Acceptance for Vegetarian Diets

Epigraph: Margaret Visser, "The Sins of the Flesh," *Granta* 52 (Winter 1995): 113–131, quotation on page 129.
1. C. Arthur, "Meatless Menus Rising at Restaurants," *American Demographics* 14, no. 2 (1992): 18.
2. Nancy Chapman, "Where Is the Soyfood Market Headed?" *Third Annual Soyfoods Symposium Proceedings* (Louisville, K.Y.: 1998), pp. 21–25.
3. Laura Cuthbert, "Convenience and Taste Boost Frozen Sales," *Natural Foods Merchandiser*, March 1998 (available on-line at www.newhope.com/nfm-online).
4. Ibid.
5. "Expanding Markets," *Natural Foods Merchandiser*, April 1998 (available on-line at www.newhope.com/nfm-online).
6. Peter Goldbitz, "Meat Alternative Sales Sizzling," *Natural Foods Merchandiser*, January 1996 (available on-line at www.newhope.com/nfm-online); Cuthbert, "Convenience and Taste Boost Frozen Sales."
7. Rekha Balu and Vanessa O'Connell, "Gardenburger's Big Advertising Campaign May Boost Worthington's Sales," *Wall Street Journal*, May 20, 1998, p. B8.
8. Laura Cuthbert, "Soyfoods Sales Surge with More Products and New Customers," *Natural Foods Merchandiser*, February 1998 (available on-line at www.newhope.com/nfm-online).
9. Amy Rosenbaum Clark, "Carrot and Stick," *Vegetarian Times* (April 1995): 109; for further discussion about why tofu often inspires such loathing, see Donna Maurer, "Tofu and Taste: Explicating the Relationships between Food, Language, and Embodiment," *Humanity and Society* 20, no. 3 (August 1996): 61–76.
10. Cuthbert, "Soyfoods Sales Surge."
11. "U.S. Allows More Vegetable Protein in School Menus" (Reuters syndicated article), March 9, 2000.
12. "School Kids 'Grade' Soy-Enhanced Entrees," *Food Service Director* 9, no. 11 (1996): 12.

13. "U.S. Allows More Vegetable Protein in School Menus."

14. Ibid.

15. "Dairy Group Has a Cow Over 'Milk' That Isn't" (*Washington Post* syndicated article), *Watertown Daily Times,* March 5, 2000, pp. E1–E2.

16. Mary Grauerholz, "Veggie Heaven: Restaurants Making It Easy to Go Meatless," *Boston Globe,* August 13, 2000, p. C3.

17. "Note from the Contributors," *Vegetarian Journal* 19 (May–June 2000): 1.

18. Janice Matsumoto, "Garden Plates," *Restaurants and Institutions* (April 1998): 58–64.

19. Toni Lydecker, "Veg Out," *Restaurant Business* 97, no. 5 (1998): 68–78.

20. Alan Beardsworth, "The Management of Food Ambivalence: Erosion and Reconstruction?" in *Eating Agendas: Food and Nutrition as Social Problems,* ed. Donna Maurer and Jeffery Sobal, pp. 117–142 (Hawthorne, N.Y.: Aldine de Gruyter, 1995).

21. Matsumoto, "Garden Plates."

22. Margaret Visser, "The Sins of the Flesh," *Granta* 52 (Winter 1995): 113–131. 23. Mark Hamstra, "Quick-Serve Operators Continue Their Quest to Provide Fast, Flavorful Low-Fat Fare," *Nation's Restaurant News,* September 28, 1998, pp. 45–48.

24. Carole Sugarman, "Fast-Food Chains Expand Veggie Options," *Washington Post,* March 25, 1998, p. G1.

25. "Lynchburg College Adds Veggie Option," *Food Service Director,* March 15, 1997, p. 6.

26. Jeff Hirschfeld, "Adding More Ethnic Options," *Food Service Director* 9, no. 3 (1996): 114.

27. Donna Boss and Karolyn Schuster, "A Balance of Tastes," *Food Management* 30, no. 10 (1995): 74–88.

28. Alan Beardsworth and Teresa Keil, "Contemporary Vegetarianism in the U.K.: Challenge and Incorporation?" *Appetite* 20 (1993): 229–234.

Chapter 8: What Is the Future of the Vegetarian Movement?

Epigraph: Charles Stahler, "How Many Vegetarians Are There?" *Vegetarian Journal* 12 (July–August 1994): 6–9.

1. Judy Klemesrud, "World Vegetarians Meet to Talk—and Eat," *New York Times,* August 22, 1975, pp. 36–37, quotation on p. 36.

2. In addition, some conflicts that may affect the ability of organizations to work together have recently arisen; see www.vegsource.com.

3. Peter Ibarra and John I. Kitsuse, "Vernacular Constituents of Moral Discourse: An Interactionist Proposal for the Study of Social Problems," in *Constructionist Controversies: Issues in Social Problems Theory*, ed. Gale Miller and James A. Holstein, pp. 21–54 (Hawthorne, N.Y.: Aldine de Gruyter, 1993), quotation on p. 35.

4. Ronald Troyer, "The Surprising Resurgence of the Smoking Problem," in *Images of Issues: Typifying Contemporary Social Problems*, 1st ed., ed. Joel Best, pp. 159–176 (Hawthorne, N.Y.: Aldine de Gruyter, 1989).

5. Field notes, International Vegan Festival, August 1995.

6. Warren Hodge, "In a Crisis, Vegetables, Not Beef, for British, *New York Times*, April 1, 2001 (available on-line at www.nytimes.com).

7. John C. Burnham, *Bad Habits: Drinking, Smoking, Taking Drugs, Gambling, Sexual Misbehavior, and Swearing in American History* (New York: New York University Press, 1983); Ronald J. Troyer and Gerald E. Markle, "Coffee Drinking: An Emerging Social Problem?" *Social Problems* 31 (1984): 403–416, especially pp. 410–411; Pierre Bourdieu, *Distinction: A Social Critique of the Judgement of Taste* (Cambridge, Mass.: Harvard University Press, 1985); Julia Twigg, "Vegetarianism and the Meanings of Meat," in *The Sociology of Food and Eating*, ed. Anne Murcott, pp. 18–30 (Aldershot, England: Gower, 1983).

8. M. L. Apte and Judith Katona-Apte, "Diet and Social Movements in American Society: The Last Two Decades," in *Food in Change: Eating Habits from the Middle Ages to the Present Day*, ed. Alexander Fenton and Eszter Kisban, pp. 26–33 (Edinburgh, Scotland: John Donald Publishers, 1986); Timothy Miller, *The Hippies and American Values* (Knoxville: University of Tennessee Press, 1991), pp. 118–119.

9. Charles Edgley and Dennis Brissett, "Health Nazis and the Cult of the Perfect Body: Some Polemical Observations," *Symbolic Interaction* 13 (1990): 257–279.

10. Warren J. Belasco, *Appetite for Change: How the Counterculture Took on the Food Industry* (Ithaca, N.Y.: Cornell University Press, 1993), p. 249.

11. See Gary L. Francione, *Rain without Thunder: The Ideology of the Animal Rights Movement* (Philadelphia: Temple University Press, 1996).

12. John D. McCarthy and Mayer Zald, "Resource Mobilization and Social Movements: A Partial Theory," *American Journal of Sociology* 82 (1976): 1212–1241; Myra Marx Ferree and Frederick D. Miller, "Mobilization and Meaning: Toward an Integration of Social Psychological and Resource Perspectives on Social Movements," *Sociological Inquiry* 55 (1985): 38–61; Kurt Back and Margaret Glasgow, "Social Networks and

Psychological Conditions in Dietary Preferences: Gourmets and Vegetarians," *Basic and Applied Social Psychology* 2 (1981): 1–9; Pasi Falk, *The Consuming Body* (London: Sage, 1994); Benjamin D. Zablocki and Rosabeth Moss Kanter, "The Differentiation of Life-Styles," *Annual Review of Sociology* 2 (1976): 269–298.

13. McCarthy and Zald, "Resource Mobilization and Social Movements."

Select Bibliography

This listing includes social scientific books and articles and general interest books that may be of special interest to the reader.

Adams, Carol. *The Sexual Politics of Meat: A Feminist-Vegetarian Critical Theory.* New York: Continuum, 1991.

Akers, Keith. *A Vegetarian Sourcebook: The Nutrition, Ecology, and Ethics of a Natural Foods Diet.* Arlington, Va.: Vegetarian Press, 1983.

Amato, Paul, and Sonia Partridge. *The New Vegetarians: Promoting Health and Protecting Life.* New York: Plenum, 1989.

Back, Kurt, and Margaret Glasgow. "Social Networks and Psychological Conditions in Dietary Preferences: Gourmets and Vegetarians." *Basic and Applied Social Psychology* 2 (1981): 1–9.

Barkas, Janet. *The Vegetable Passion.* New York: Charles Scribner's Sons, 1975.

Beardsworth, Alan, and Teresa Keil. "Contemporary Vegetarianism in the U.K.: Challenge and Incorporation?" *Appetite* 20 (1993): 229–234.

———. "The Vegetarian Option: Varieties, Conversions, Motives, and Careers." *Sociological Review* 40 (1992): 253–293.

Belasco, Warren J. *Appetite for Change: How the Counterculture Took on the Food Industry.* Ithaca, N.Y.: Cornell University Press, 1993.

Carson, Gerald. *Cornflake Crusade.* New York: Rinehart, 1957.

Cooper, Charles K., Thomas N. Wise, and Lee S. Mann. "Psychological and Cognitive Characteristics of Vegetarians." *Psychosomatics* 26, no. 6 (1985): 521–527.

Delahoyde, Michael, and Susan C. Despenich. "Creating Meat-Eaters: The Child as Advertising Target." *Journal of Popular Culture* 28, no. 1 (1994): 135–149.

Dietz, Thomas, Ann Stirling Frisch, Linda Lalof, Paul C. Stern, and Gregory A. Guagnano. "Values and Vegetarianism: An Exploratory Analysis." *Rural Sociology* 60, no. 3 (1995): 533–542.

Dombrowski, Daniel A. *Vegetarianism: The Philosophy behind the Diet.* Wellingborough, England: Thorsons, 1985.

Dwyer, Johanna, Laura D.V.H. Dwyer, Kathryn Dowd, Randy Frances Kandel, and Jean Mayer. "The New Vegetarians: The Natural High?" *Journal of the American Dietetic Association* 65 (1974): 529–536.

Dwyer, Johanna, Laura Mayer, Randy F. Kandel, and Jean Mayer. "The New Vegetarians: Who Are They?" *Journal of the American Dietetic Association* 62 (1973): 503–509.

Fiddes, Nick. "Declining Meat: Past, Present . . . and Future Imperfect?" In *Food, Health and Identity*, ed. Pat Caplan, pp. 252–266. New York: Routledge, 1997.

———. *Meat: A Natural Symbol*. London: Routledge, 1991.

Fox, Michael Allen. *Deep Vegetarianism*. Philadelphia: Temple University Press, 1999.

Freeland-Graves, Jeanne H., Sue Greninger, Glenn R. Graves, and Robert K. Young. "Health Practices, Attitudes, and Beliefs of Vegetarians and Nonvegetarians." *Journal of the American Dietetic Association* 86 (1986): 913–918.

Freeland-Graves, Jeanne H., Sue Greninger, and Robert K. Young. "A Demographic and Social Profile of Age- and Sex-Matched Vegetarians and Nonvegetarians." *Journal of the American Dietetic Association* 86 (1986): 907–913.

Gvion-Rosenberg, Liora. "Why Do Vegetarian Restaurants Serve Hamburgers? Toward an Understanding of a Cuisine." *Semiotica* 80, nos. 1–2 (1990): 61–79.

Hamilton, Malcolm. "Eating Ethically: 'Spiritual' and 'Quasi-religious' Aspects of Vegetarianism." *Journal of Contemporary Religion* 15 (2000): 65–83.

Havala, Suzanne. *The Complete Idiot's Guide to Being Vegetarian*. New York: Macmillan, 1999.

Jabs, Jennifer, Carol M. Devine, and Jeffery Sobal. "Maintaining Vegetarian Diets: Personal Factors, Social Networks and Environmental Resources." *Canadian Journal of Dietetic Practice and Research* 59, no. 4 (1998): 183–189.

———. "Model of the Process of Adopting Vegetarian Diets: Health Vegetarians and Ethical Vegetarians." *Journal of Nutrition Education* 30 (1998): 196–202.

Jabs, Jennifer, Jeffery Sobal, and Carol M. Devine. "Managing Vegetarianism: Identities, Norms, and Interactions." *Ecology of Food and Nutrition* 39 (2000): 375–394.

Kim, Esther H., Karen M. Schroeder, Robert F. Houser Jr., and Johanna T. Dwyer. "Two Small Surveys, Twenty-five Years Apart, Investigating Motivations of Dietary Choice in Two Groups of Vegetarians in the

Boston Area." *Journal of the American Dietetic Association* 99, no. 5 (1999): 598–601.

Krizmanic, Judy. *A Teen's Guide to Going Vegetarian.* New York: Puffin Books, 1994.

Lappé, Frances Moore. *Diet for a Small Planet.* New York: Ballentine, 1971.

Lyman, Howard, with Glen Merzer. *Mad Cowboy: Plain Truth from the Cattle Rancher Who Won't Eat Meat.* New York: Charles Scribner's Sons, 1998.

MacNair, Rachel. "The Psychology of Becoming a Vegetarian." *Vegetarian Nutrition* 2 (1998): 96–102.

Marcus, Erik. *Vegan: The New Ethics of Eating.* Ithaca, N.Y.: McBooks Press, 1998.

Maurer, Donna. "Meat as a Social Problem: Rhetorical Strategies in the Contemporary Vegetarian Literature." In *Eating Agendas: Food and Nutrition as Social Problems,* ed. Donna Maurer and Jeffery Sobal, pp. 143–163. Hawthorne, N.Y.: Aldine de Gruyter, 1995.

———. "Too Skinny or Vibrant and Healthy? Weight Management in the Vegetarian Movement." In *Weighty Issues: Fatness and Thinness as Social Problems,* ed. Jeffery Sobal and Donna Maurer, pp. 209–229. Hawthorne, N.Y.: Aldine de Gruyter, 1999.

———. "The Vegetarian Movement in North America: An Examination of Movement Culture and Collective Strategy." Ph.D. diss., Carbondale: Southern Illinois University, 1997.

McKenzie, John. "Profile on Vegans." *Plant Foods in Human Nutrition* 2, no. 2 (1971): 79–88.

Melina, Vesanto, Brenda Davis, and Victoria Harrison. *Becoming Vegetarian: The Complete Guide to Adopting a Healthy Vegetarian Diet.* Summertown, Tenn.: Book Publishing, 1995.

Moran, Victoria. *Compassion: The Ultimate Ethic.* Wellingborough, England: Thorsons, 1985.

Nissenbaum, Stephen. *Sex, Diet, and Debility in Jacksonian America: Sylvester Graham and Health Reform.* Westport, Conn.: Greenwood Press, 1980.

Ossipow, Lawrence. "Vegetarianism and Fatness: An Undervalued Perception of the Body." In *The Social Aspects of Obesity,* ed. I. de Garine and N. J. Pollack, pp. 127–143. Luxembourg, Belgium: Gordon and Breach, 1995.

Powell, Kimberly D. "Lifestyle as a Dimension of Social Movement Study: A Case Study of the Vegetarian Movement in the United States." Ph.D. diss., Department of Speech Communications, University of Georgia, 1992.

Richardson, N. J., R. Shepherd, and N. Elliman. "Meat Consumption, Definition of Meat and Trust in Information Sources in the UK Population and the Members of the Vegetarian Society." *Ecology of Food and Nutrition* 33 (1994): 1–13.

Robbins, John. *Diet for a New America.* Waltham, Mass.: Stillpoint, 1987.

Rozin, Paul, Maureen Markwith, and Caryn Stoess. "Moralization and Becoming a Vegetarian: The Transformation of Preferences into Values and the Recruitment of Disgust." *Psychological Science* 8, no. 2 (1997): 67–73.

Sims, Laura. "Food-Related Value-Orientations, Attitudes, and Beliefs of Vegetarians and Non-vegetarians." *Ecology of Food and Nutrition* 7 (1977): 23–35.

Singer, Peter. *Animal Liberation: A New Ethic for Our Treatment of Animals.* New York: Avon, 1975.

Spencer, Colin. *The Heretic's Feast: A History of Vegetarianism.* Hanover, N.H.: University Press of New England, 1995.

Stepaniak, Joanne. *The Vegan Sourcebook.* Los Angeles: Lowell House, 1998.

Twigg, Julia. "Food for Thought: Purity and Vegetarianism." *Religion* 9 (1979): 13–35.

———. "Vegetarianism and the Meanings of Meat." In *The Sociology of Food and Eating,* ed. Anne Murcott, pp. 18–30. Aldershot, England: Gower, 1983.

Visser, Margaret. "The Sins of the Flesh." *Granta* 52 (Winter 1995): 113–131.

West, Eric D. "The Psychological Health of Vegans Compared with Two Other Groups." *Plant Foods and Human Nutrition* 2 (1972): 147–149.

White, Randall F., Jennifer Seymour, and Erica Frank. "Vegetarianism among US Women Physicians." *Journal of the American Dietetic Association* 99, no. 5 (1999): 595–598.

Whorton, James. *Crusaders for Fitness: The History of American Health Reformers.* Princeton, N.J.: Princeton University Press, 1982.

Worsley, Anthony and Grace Skrzypiec. "Teenage Vegetarianism: Beauty or the Beast?" *Nutrition Research* 17, no. 3 (1997): 391–404.

Yntema, Sharon K. *Vegetarian Children: A Supportive Guide for Parents.* Ithaca, N.Y.: McBooks Press, 1987.

Index

187